Contesting Colonial Authority

Contesting Colonial Authority

Medicine and Indigenous Responses in Nineteenth- and Twentieth-Century India

Edited by Poonam Bala

LEXINGTON BOOKS
Lanham • Boulder • New York • Toronto • Plymouth, UK

Published by Lexington Books
A wholly owned subsidiary of The Rowman & Littlefield Publishing Group, Inc.
4501 Forbes Boulevard, Suite 200, Lanham, Maryland 20706
www.rowman.com

10 Thornbury Road, Plymouth PL6 7PP, United Kingdom

British Library Cataloguing in Publication Information Available

Library of Congress Cataloging-in-Publication Data
Contesting colonial authority : medicine and indigenous responses in nineteenth- and twentieth-century India / edited by Poonam Bala.
p. ; cm.
Includes bibliographical references and index.
ISBN 978-0-7391-7023-6 (cloth : alk. paper)—ISBN 978-0-7391-7024-3 (electronic)
I. Bala, Poonam. [DNLM: 1. History of Medicine—India. 2. Culture—India. 3. Government—India. 4. History, 19th Century—India. 5. History, 20th Century—India. WZ 70 JI4]
610.954'09034—dc23
2012001467

The paper used in this publication meets the minimum requirements of American National Standard for Information Sciences Permanence of Paper for Printed Library Materials, ANSI/NISO Z39.48-1992.

Printed in the United States of America

Dedicated to my father (late), Raghubir Narain, for inspiring in me a passion for history, and my mother, Sharda, for her love and support at all times.

Contents

Acknowledgments

I would like to thank all the authors of respective chapters in this volume for their contributions, patience, and prompt responses during various stages of editing this work, which went a long way in making this volume feasible. I should also like to express my appreciation to my colleague, Phil Manning at the Department of Sociology, Cleveland State University, for providing a collegial work environment and the necessary facilities required for scholarly productivity. Thanks are also due to Phyllis Smith and Gloria Watson in the Sociology Department, for their help and kindness, and to Glenda Carbaugh in the Economics Department (all at Cleveland State University) for her support. I am also grateful to the staff at the Kelvin Smith Library at Case Western Reserve University, the Allen Memorial Medical Library, and Cleveland State University and the Ratan Tata Library (Delhi), for their help in procuring the required research material. To John Grabowski and Alan Rocke at Case Western Reserve University, I am especially grateful for an enabling support in the use of various resources. I also offer my thanks to Neelam Gupta and Meera Kak for their support during my brief visits to India. I would also like to thank Erin Walpole for her help during the editorial process and Stephanie Brooks for her immense patience in the final production stages of this volume (at Rowman & Littlefield Publishing Group, respectively).

Finally, a special note of gratitude to my mother, Sharda, for providing the much-needed support, care, and above all, an inspiration for a continued zeal for academic pursuits.

—Poonam Bala
Cleveland
February 2012

Introduction

Poonam Bala

Indian encounters with Western medicine and colonial imperatives produced new forms of structures, which I would call "paradigms of defense" within which trajectories of negotiation between Indian and Western knowledge could be perceived. Concomitantly, Indian responses to colonial imperatives are to be seen in terms of these paradigms or mechanisms of "defense" which emerged primarily from the said encounters with policy dictates. They were more akin to apparatuses of covert resistance created when colonial demands for reform to modernity required regressions from traditional forms of knowledge and practice. With the emergence of new structural paradigms, thus, new frameworks within which Indian medical knowledge could be more readily identified and negotiated and made accessible in the changing socio-political contexts, became apparent. This also entailed development of new "spatial technologies of health, in the form of a new set of relations"[1] within which new contesting relations between knowledge and colonial policies were visible.

A note on the use of the terms *authority* and *contestation*: while authority has been understood in terms of ideologies of the colonial empire, it also indicates hegemonic ideologies, as observed by Engles and Marks in their noteworthy study on ideas of hegemony and the colonial state in India and Africa. Their study brings out the limitations of hegemonic strategies of the colonial state owing to its transitional character and its contradictory identity as Mughal successor state on the one hand and rational modernizer on the other. Even when adopting the second role, the colonial state's hegemonic aspirations were compromised, for not every effort to gain consent could be described as an attempt to gain hegemony.[2] Gauging by this definition, colonial authority can be perceived as being limited in gaining complete authority in India. However, for our purpose, what is significant is not the success or failure of the colonial imperatives in gaining social and political preeminence, but the outcome of these as they unfolded to form new structures for negotiation of traditional forms of knowledge. Thus, while the colonial state had to justify and legitimize its rule in India, through "the demonstration of an excess of power, the theatrical representation of the utter superiority and inviolability of imperial authority,"[3] it also adopted various means of "appropriating 'traditional' signs of authority."[4] Various alliances were formed as a result between the traditional sections of the Indian population and the colonial state alliances which also facilitated extensions of hegemonic power directed toward "transforming indigenous tradition into the universal forms of a rational and scientifically ordered social life."[5] The chapters in this volume focus on the paradigms and structures that were formed as a result of these alliances which also formed sites where hegemonic claims could be contested by indigenous authorities. These sites also indicate a gradual "institutionalization of rational—bureaucratic norms—," norms that were to be extended to colonized population in order to be firmly embedded.[6]

In understanding issues around power and power relations, thus, ideas of contestation remain paramount. While alliances with the colonial hegemony may indicate "consent," as linked to Gramsci's notion of hegemony, they gradually withered away as the small section of the educated intelligentsia and colonized elite emerged as the agency through which the "external force of the colonial critique of indigenous tradition turned into an internal critique."[7] Foucault describes them as not always prohibitive for they tend to traverse and produce things, induce pleasure, forms of knowledge, and produce discourse."[8]

While issues of power and hegemony enabling an understanding of the trajectories of conformity and resistance to Western medicine and colonial imperatives in India have been discussed at length in several scholarly writings, this volume portrays various indigenous and subaltern responses of the Indian population to "subvert" or counteract colonial policies toward the existing forms of medical knowledge. While revisiting Indian medicine, how did these responses alter the outlook on Indian medical knowledge and practice? How were they viewed by the Indian elites, by the nationalists and by the rest of the Indian population in their move to revisit and frame a new social character of Indian medicine—creating new structures of institutions, marketing, public health, and of scientization? These are pending pertinent questions answers to which can be gauged from the chapters in this volume. They focus on indigenous interpretations and mechanisms through which Indian medicine was projected against the cultural background of a rich medical tradition in nineteenth- and early twentieth-century colonial India—either as nationalists, medical practitioners, reformers, or as part of the general public. This volume brings together various forms of contestational strategies which produced paradigms of "defense." To explain the theoretical framework within which these chapters have been written, I have used Kuhn's notion of paradigms that explain a theoretical framework within which ideas are to be perceived.[9] This volume brings together chapters that focus on colonial India during the late nineteenth and early twentieth centuries. Generally, while Asia's encounter with medicine and colonial imperatives produced "particular vocabularies and frameworks through which cultures and communities could be identified, categorized, and transformed into accessible knowledge," the history of colonial Burma (then a significant part of British-ruled India) reveals that the administrative connection to India might have corresponded to the manner in which healing culture was conceptualized. Due to changing political circumstances surrounding the question of Burma's separation from India, the image of traditional medicine shifted to represent a distinct form of Burmese criminality and resistance.[10] This provides new understandings on the extent of influence of the empire, not often discussed in medical history discourses which would complement the main arguments. Yet, another dimension in the volume is enriched by a discussion on colonial Goa that enriches our discussion by providing new dimensions on how elites were instrumental in establishing their demands for Western medical education and practice in colonial Goa.

In a move to construct a national and cultural identity during the height of the national movement in colonial India, and coeval with anti-British sentiments, indigenous medicine formed an essential component of the overall political prerogatives of "rejuvenating" the pristine heritage of India. Poonam Bala discusses these prerogatives to highlight issues involved in engaging Ayurveda as a model of indigenous power and authority. These issues became visible at a time when a general disbelief in colonial policies as being detrimental to all existing forms of knowledge prevailed in the minds of the Indian people. Bala examines the process by which medical encounter and the national movement in colonial India led to changes in indigenous paradigms and identity reconstructed through modernizing and reform missions. This happened at a time when education in indigenous sciences was not a prioritized agenda of the colonial imperatives. While medical institutions and organizations are a powerful means of shaping as well as preserving the traditional identity of cultural expressions, claims to possession of "indigeneity," thus, displayed political undertones that validated different forms of knowledge in colonial India. Shamshad Khan, in a similar respect, examines the various ambiguities within the nationalist discourse on medicine and health and within conforming patterns of indigenous traditions. He also demonstrates that efforts to revitalize Indian systems of medicine were not devoid of internal differences which were intricately entangled with class, communal, religious, and political agendas.

While the introduction of Western medicine as an administrative exigency justified the paradigm of power and cultural hegemony, the rise of the Indian pharmaceuticals and the medical market marked an important transition in the way medical practice was to be channelized in later years; the rise of the printing press provided further impetus to the popularity of indigenous drugs, facilitating a new social identity to Indian medicine. In response to imperial policies toward indigenous drugs, there was a move toward commodification and commercialization of indigenous drugs so that they could be made more marketable to the public at large, despite a curious display of "romantic" association and antagonism between state ideologies and power in previous years. Madhulika Banerjee frames her argument within the social parameters of class consciousness and responsibilities to understand how the middle class used their familiarity with Western social and political thoughts to promulgate the popularity of Indian drugs. Following partly from the economic and industrial developments in the European world, as also from the competing Western market for drugs, the production of indigenous drugs on a large scale by local elites, scientists, and nationalists, seemed imperative. The growth of the middle class and the economic, political, and social changes in the country were sure indicators of this change.

Medical education at the Medical School of Goa, a Portuguese colonial institution, is exemplary of the outcome of the local groups who adopted Western medicine in order to strengthen their own political agendas under colonial rule. Cristiana Bastos highlights the main issues around the Medical School of Goa and indigenous involvement in keeping the institution functional, despite colonial attempts at abolishing it.

While medical education, on the one hand, forged relations and cooperation between colonial administration and the Indian educated middle class, on the other it proved inimical to the stability of the colonial rule by challenging its medical policies and innovations. What happened when medical education was made available to the urban elite of Indian society? What became apparent were the structural changes in medical education with the rapid Indianization of the IMS (Indian Medical Service), especially at the turn of the twentieth century, when new opportunities for Western-educated Indian practitioners, and the emergence of the Indian middle class made the strength of the indigenous groups more prominent. Between 1860 and 1920, political changes in India, the rapid spread of English education, as also establishment of medical schools by indigenous practitioners and rich elites, "subverted" British attempts to use medical education for their officers and the army, for training in Western ideals had rendered easy realization of "colonial intents" in India by the educated elites. The introduction of the English language as the medium of instruction in 1835 opened up new strategies of encounters with the Indian population. Nevertheless, the existence of Indian vernaculars and their patronage remained an area of concern for indigenous authorities. Shrimoy Roy Chaudhury examines these issues in the light of the emergence of *daktari* as a vernacular idiom of therapeutic agency, representing it as a natural medical intervention on the bodies of native subjects.

The issue of providing health services to women in colonial India was an important offshoot of British policies that engaged new perspectives on gender issues and the practice of medicine in the context of colonialism.[11] The political edge to the Dufferin Fund lay in an overt rejection of traditional *dais* midwives, and the preference for Western-trained European doctors to handle issues of maternity and child health. While the Dufferin Fund often aroused native suspicion about its intentions, the nationalist perspectives reified its indispensability in such matters. Yet, the Fund existed as a manifestation of the alleged superiority of colonial ideologies of politics, gender relations, and health. Seán Lang uses political parameters to analyze some issues central to our understanding of the impact of the Dufferin Fund. Although, occasionally punctuated by native resistance, it represented an area in which Indian opinions on employment of Indian women doctors were of prime concern, especially after their exclusion from higher posts of the government. This, then, was resistance at its best, for Indians aspired to control the administration of the Fund.

A prolonged scarcity of indigenous female professionals in medicine, midwifery, and nursing was a result of lack of colonial interest in medical education and employment of women doctors. Atsuko Naono highlights these issues through her discussion on Lady Dufferin's Fund in Burma. Besides the Fund, several philanthropic institutions expressed interest in addressing concerns about medical education among indigenous women, as well as improving infant mortality and family. In addition, she also examines the factors that contributed to colonial discourse on the education of female medical professionals in colonial India/Burma.

The medical encounter between Unani and Western medicine was one that called for validating the present through various strategies of memory and representation. While the medical knowledge in Unani texts were left unquestioned, attempts to reaffirm their scientific authenticity remained paramount, especially during the height of the nationalist movement. While indigenous claims of the decline of traditional knowledge under colonial rule were crucial in assessing the dismantling and reformation policies of colonial rule, both Ayurveda and Unani were perceived by them as being "marginalized" as a result. The establishment of medical institutions, thus, was a means through which medical knowledge could be translated into a useful medical paradigm. Neshat Quaiser discusses issues of perceived "marginalization" in the light of Western medical absolutism and colonial representations of medical knowledge, arguing that resistance to Western absolutism found expression in reconstructing the past through memory located within the literate anticolonial sphere.

Public health under colonial India was an area of major concern for the colonial administrators, as much as it was for the civilian population and the perceived effects of the severity of the epidemics that ravaged the country. There was always a conflict between Western and traditional modes of handling diseases that existed in epidemic proportions. The success in handling major health hazards lay in active cooperation of the Indian population, although

> such cooperation was impossible in a colonial situation in which notions of racial superiority, and cultural distance made difficult constructive relations between rulers and the ruled, and in which government priorities would always favour the former.[12]

Elements of religious attributes of diseases, thus, remained paramount alongside the local systems of knowledge that became increasingly invested with a competitive agenda. Nevertheless, integration, cooperation, authority, collision, and resistance to coercive sanitary reforms were visible markers of these forms of resistance. Yet, as Arabinda Samanta has argued in his discussion on the malaria epidemic, the prophylactic measures adopted through public health experts to combat malaria met with severe opposition, disbelief, and suspicion exemplifying a "war" against bad government—a fact that throws light on the political foundations of colonial medical interventions in India and the subsequent popular resistance that was set amid caution and care. The success of public health initiatives meant a committed negotiation and involvement of the local population. Yet, indigenous response to government public health measures in the nineteenth and twentieth centuries, expressed itself in terms of suspicion and noncompliance with public health measures.

A general conclusion that may be drawn from the chapters in this volume is that the indigenous population became an active agency of understanding traditional forms of knowledge, and also of the colonial hegemonic ideologies. It became more pervious to indigenous interpretations and reinterpretations of medical thoughts. In the process, while structural forms and paradigms were framed to accommodate these new ideas, they also became a site whereby medical identity could be negotiated and altered to reach the Indian population at large. Contestations, acceptance, and resistance were obvious outcomes of these encounters, marked by alternating overt consent and covert resistance, expressed through exemplary paradigms of nationalism, medical aid, medical education, medical discourses, memory, reconstruction of the past, and prophylactic inverventions

NOTES

1. Nikolas Rose, "Medicine, History and the Present." Pp. 48–72 in *Reassessing Foucault: Power, Medicine and the Body: Power, Medicine and the Body*, edited by Collin Jones and Roy Porter (Routledge: London, 1994).

2. Dagmar Engels and Shula Marks, "Introduction: Hegemony in a Colonial Context." Pp. 1–15 in *Contesting Colonial Hegemony: State and Society in Africa and India*, edited by Dagmar Engels and Shula Marks (London: British Academic Press, 1994).

3. Partha Chatterjee, "Was there a Hegemonic Project of the Colonial State?" Pp. 79–84 in *Contesting Colonial Hegemony*.

4. Chatterjee, "Was There a Hegemonic Project?"

5. Chatterjee, "Was There a Hegemonic Project?" 83.

6. See details in Chatterjee, "Was There a Hegemonic Project?"

7. See details in Chatterjee, "Was there a Hegemonic Project?" 83.

8. M. Foucault, "Truth and Power." Pp. 117 in *Power/Knowledge: Selected Interviews and Other Writings, 1972–1977*, by M. Foucault (Brighton: Harvester, 1980).

9. See details in Thomas S. Kuhn, *The Structure of Scientific Revolutions* (Chicago: University of Chicago Press, 1996).

10. Maitrii Aung-Thwin, "Healing, Rebellion, and the Law: Ethnologies of Medicine in Colonial Burma, 1928–1932," *Journal of Burma Studies* 14 (2010): 151–85 (abstract).

11. Maneesha Lal, "The Politics of Gender and Medicine in Colonial India: The Countess of Dufferin's Fund, 1885–1888," *Bulletin of History of Medicine* 1 (1994): 29–66 (abstract).

12. Mark Harrison, *Public Health in British India: Anglo-Indian Preventive Medicine, 1859–1914* (Cambridge: Cambridge University Press), 234.

Chapter One

"Nationalizing" Medicine

The Changing Paradigm of Ayurveda in British India

Poonam Bala

Interpretations of indigenous science as a result of changing policy structures led to the creation of new structural paradigms of medical science which became a site of contestation under imperial rule in India. Although Western medicine developed an intelligible relationship with India and her culture, it was unable to sustain the bond toward the end of the nineteenth century as a result of the changing social and political climate and transformations at the time. The imperial prerogative of science, medicine, and research was, thus, contested by the nationalist visions of a celebrated past on which was premised a triumphant future. This chapter proposes to discuss two arguments. Firstly, exponents of Indian science, medicine, and culture established a new paradigm as a means to "contest" the imperial policies in nineteenth- and early twentieth-century India. Secondly, the new paradigm, a product of the national movement, formed a new *medico-cultural identity* for Indian medicine—an identity that would successfully claim the professional and scientific status of medicine in postcolonial India.

PERCEPTIONS AND COLONIAL ATTITUDES

The new paradigm of a "nationalized" medicine altered the course of medical knowledge and practice in colonial and postcolonial India. The earlier attempts of "bringing India and its newly discovered arts, sciences and history into a closer and more intelligible relationship with Western knowledge"[1] were replaced by the emerging awareness of science, medicine and their practical advantages.

To follow the argument of a paradigm, and to understand the trajectory of medical practice, this chapter utilizes the Kuhnian notion of paradigms. In building a new understanding of Ayurveda, different attitudes were adopted not only by the exponents of Ayurveda but also by Western medicine and its practitioners. It was more pertinent for the latter to understand and assimilate the medical knowledge that was already popular and entrenched in Indian society and culture. In Kuhn's definition, assimilation of knowledge and theory "requires the reconstruction of prior theory and the reevaluation of prior fact."[2] This perception of validating the past was a route to "normal science," which meant that a recognition of India and her achievements was premised on research that was

> firmly based upon one or more past scientific achievement, achievements that some particular scientific community acknowledges for a time as supplying the foundation for its further practice.[3]

While, in the early part of the nineteenth century, an attitude of indifference and noninterference by the Company rulers prevailed, there was a general feeling that any attempts at interfering with social and cultural ideologies of the people of India would likely result in disagreements and extreme popular reactions. This attitude found expression in the initial policies of accommodation of local practitioners trained in indigenous medicine. Besides, attempts were also made to employ them as subordinate health workers in hospitals, primarily staffed by British physicians,[4] with the skilled ones promoted as native doctors in regiments and civil stations.

NEW IDENTITY AND INDIAN RESPONSES

The quest for an identity by the proponents of Ayurveda and Unani was, by no measure, an indication of the efficacy or perception of a "failed" science and scientific practice. On the contrary, the move to locate Indian medicine in a new political climate justified claims to a "progressive" science requiring attention of a different kind—attention that would focus on proving the scientific existence hitherto unrecognized by the administrators. Thus, in a move to reassess and construct a national cultural identity during the height of the national movement in colonial India, coeval with disbelief in British rule, Indian forms of knowledge, including Ayurveda and Unani, formed an essential component of the overall political prerogatives of claims over a rich historical past. Here then follows an account of the trajectory of engaging indigenous medical knowledge as a viable model of indigenous power and authority in an attempt to establish a recognized medical and social space within the changing political milieu.

It is widely known that despite the changing attitude toward indigenous forms of knowledge (represented by Ayurveda and Unani), and the withdrawal of British State support to indigenous medical institutions and practitioners in the nineteenth century, the former continued to build a clientele and popular support. Nevertheless, the growing differences between the development in medical knowledge and practice of British-borne Western medicine and indigenous forms of knowledge, coupled with the changing nature of government policies acted as a precursor to various conflicts and instability in India in later years. Issues of creating a medical identity, an independent medical profession, and seeking state support, thus, became an apparent outcome of these transformations.

The real, and initial, blow to Indian medical practitioners came with the abolition of the Native Medical Institution in 1824 for its "inability" to meet the stipulated requirements of a successful medical practice of anatomy and surgery. While the reasons for the change in medical policy at this stage may have been apparent in terms of the scientific validity, they were not limited to these. The Native Exclusion Act of 1791 and the move toward "alien solutions" to problems in Indian society and culture defined the much-vaunted English administrative machinery that formed colonial ideas of "producing an elite of acculturated Englishmen."[5] James Mill's controversial book, *The History of British India*, however, was largely influential in the way policies were structured and implemented during the early years of Company rule, and was a major force behind the consolidation of Company rule. Not only did it prove inimical to favorable social and cultural policies, but it also provided a framework within which a prospective course of action was to be visualized and implemented, and the way British engagement with India was to be perceived. Mill's utilitarian inclinations inspired Thomas Babington Macaulay to "project an India based on English culture."[6] This found expression when William Bentinck as the new governor-general, in his communication with Mill, remarked, "I am going to British India but I shall not be Governor-General. It is you that will be Governor-General."[7]

The early part of the twentieth century was a turning point in the historical trajectories of the medical encounter under British rule for it laid open a popular belief and recognition of colonial policies as detrimental to indigenous science and medicine, as well as Indian culture and her traditions. In our discussion of the medical encounter, the nationalist reconstruction of the past and the subsequent quest for an identity remain paramount. As new medical paradigms and methods of understanding disease began to influence medical practice in the Western medical world, issues of professionalization of Indian medicine came to the fore. The perceived differences in Western Europe's scientific and material growth appeared to validate the scientific supremacy. While much of the civilizing prerogative could be justified as a result, with new perceptions of reverence for the medical knowledge of the ancient Hindus and its cultural links and a rich historical heritage, debates that questioned the veracity of Indian knowledge were met with opposition from the native population. Thus, the move to resuscitate Ayurveda could be seen as a part of the rising national consciousness among the Indians that sought to revive the Indian vernaculars, according prominence to the revival of Sanskrit language and literature; the latter was said to represent the perennial fount from which the vernaculars of India were derived.[8] One of the main assumptions of Hindu cultural nationalism was the belief in a religious and racial unity of the Hindus; similarly, claims of the superiority of the Vedic knowledge of the Aryans were a force behind these perceptions.[9] Constant efforts were then made to popularize India's heritage to vindicate the superiority of indigenous culture and tradition against the perceived civilizing mission of Europe.

The history of the national movement in India and the engagement of Ayurveda is, thus, a history of negotiating cultural identities of the "East" and the "West." It was also a political movement that was defined by a "mingling of old ideas with the new."[10] It was a relationship of coercion and persuasion; a relationship of coercion and accommodation that inspired the formation of a national medical culture—a new paradigm within which medical forms of knowledge and politics could be validated and combined to produce a new tradition that complied with popular and nationalistic ideals of a positive self-image. The idea of India as a nation was, thus, propelled by her unity in terms of a common history, culture, and language, all of which led to subsequent expressions of social, cultural, political, and economic nationalism.

The series of events that took place between 1905 and 1909 altered the political situation in the country with a spur in general disbelief and hostility toward the British rule. In India, while issues of identity and difference emerged as the British established the imperial administration, the rise of the anti-imperialist movement was a gradual outcome of the contradictions between the imperatives of colonial policy and the basic interests of a large number of classes and social groups in India.[11] The growth of national consciousness, as a corollary to Hindu cultural nationalism, was premised on the recognition of the degeneration of India's culture and traditions subsequent to Western colonial thoughts and practices. Hindu nationalists also visualized a cultural unity and a "modern Indian nation,"[12] often bound by aspirations of political liberalism.

Nationalism located its own subjectivity in the spiritual domain of culture, where it considered itself superior to the West and, hence, undominated and sovereign. It could not permit an encroachment by the colonial power in that domain.[13] The feeling of cultural nationalism was vehemently expressed in repeated calls for maintaining synonymity between the national movement and cultural revivalism. Along with the cultural nationalism of the movement, there also was the fact that British rule became the major cause of India's economic backwardness. The Indians, recognizing that imperialism was a barrier to the general development, felt and bewailed the economic exploitation of the country.[14] Bholanath Chandra and Chandra Nath Bose were among the prominent advocates of economic nationalism, striving assiduously for the subversion of British policy.[15] In addition to the economic and cultural nationalist doctrines, there were calls for contesting the prevailing doctrines of the political environment, for there was a widespread belief that "as subjects of the same sovereign, all Indians enjoyed common rights and privileges."[16] Political nationalism then laid down the necessity of securing power of control over provincial affairs.

Yet another factor contributing to the growth and intensification of the national movement in India was the introduction of the English language as the medium of instruction and the spread of English-style Western education in all disciplines throughout the country. English was declared as the official language making it imperative for it to be a medium through which the knowledge of English literature was to be disseminated. Mass education in English was considered impracticable because of the limited funds earmarked for educational purposes, at least that was the laid-down policy of the British administrators. Also, increasing commercial relations with the British also convinced the local population that their success in these required proficiency in the English language.

While English education intensified the nature of cultural nationalism, it led to conflicting situations between the Indians and the rulers, precipitated by the spread of foreign-oriented education among the people whose institutions, customs, and traditions were profoundly different from those of the former. Although the middle of the nineteenth century saw British interest in primary and secondary education in the Indian vernaculars, it also had an obvious impact in creating a new class of English-speaking Indian elite confined to Calcutta, Bombay, and Madras—the erstwhile presidencies of British India. As influential social groups, the Western-educated elite Indians were quick enough in responding to nationalist calls for support to Indian knowledge, for Western education had enabled them to understand Western ideologies, culture, and political thought in a more definitive manner. Thus,

> they formed voluntary associations on British lines, with paid memberships, bylaws, regular meetings, and fund-raising drives. These associations proliferated in the second half of the nineteenth century, and it is sometimes said that after 1858, they replaced armed resistance as the primary Indian response to British dominance.[17]

Ideas of new value-formation and the appeal of Enlightenment ideals almost became a necessity and an inevitable part of the new outlook of the nationalists. As a result, the rising intelligentsia formed a strong support base for the nationalist feelings prevalent at the time. Equally active were Ayurvedic enthusiasts, who were equally aware and powerful in understanding their culture and customs in a troubled economic and political milieu of the country. Thus, the recognition that contemporary traditional practices do not reflect the significant achievements of the ancient civilization as a result of their decline, due to the imposition of an alien culture that created a demand for state patronage or governmental interference from new regimes for their resuscitation, identifies most of the revivalist movements in South Asian history.[18] It may be argued that the civilizing mission of Western Europe lay open a new arena which was perceived as difficult for its Western counterpart, emphasizing that

> the virtues that the colonizers valorized through the civilizing mission ideology were overwhelmingly bourgeois. Besides, ideas of progress in science, systematic scientific inquiry, industriousness and adaptability were all hallmarks of the capitalist industrial order.[19]

Apart from the specifics of the impact of colonial policies and their impact on the native population, the feelings of general discontentment were rampant, noticeably on issues of high taxes and the increasing restrictions on the entry of educated Indians into the British civil services. Admittedly, nationalism took the form of organized resistance—organized on the belief and idea of "India of national self-determination."[20] One of the ways in which ideas of self-determination were perpetuated was in rediscovering the scientific essentials of Indian medicine. Thus, attempts to recapitulate the medical texts *Caraka Samhita* and *Susruta Samhita* (on which was based medical knowledge and practice of Ayurveda) provided new structures within which could be traced a new identity for Ayurveda as well as for Indian culture. These were also representations of

> establishing claims for the validity and rationality of Hindu science as a whole, and Ayurvedic medicine could be seen as having a practical value in the modern age and having insights and pharmacological knowledge that Western medicine had still to uncover.[21]

While Western medicine and its advocates did much to gain professional authority and preeminence with the newly developing scientific and medical outlook in medical practice, new insights into revivalism of Ayurveda were provided through public dissemination of medical knowledge. Bhagvat Sinhji's publication in 1895, *Aryan Medical Science*, was the first major defense of Indian knowledge, as also perhaps, "a noted contribution to the revivalist movement."[22]

If the concept of subjectivity were to find a place at this point of our discussion, it would mean talking about it at two levels: one, at the level of the colonial system, and the other at the level of the colonized. Fanon treats subjectivity of the colonized as being formed and shaped by the colonial system.[23] Fanon calls this aspect as "dehumanizing" which for him, is not simply a "fictional hope trope to satisfy the prejudices of the colonizing and justify their presence"[24] in another country, which Spivak would like to believe that "the colonized were obliged to occupy the space of the imperialists' self-consolidating other."[25]

INDIAN NATIONALISTS AND THE REVIVAL OF AYURVEDA

The political nature of colonialism laid the foundation of a new cultural paradigm that was by no means secular marked by a quest for a new identity. Overpowering as this may seem, the new structural and cultural paradigm of Indian medicine also reinforced the conditions that fueled the intensity of the growing nationalist ideas in the late nineteenth and early twentieth centuries. This found expression in the revivalist movement and with its new ideologies for defense and an appreciation of the past. The movement provided a cultural and political voice to the conflicts in the encounter between Indian and Western forms of knowledge.

Besides, the movement has, however, been one of major significance in Indian history. It justified claims for professional status by seeking state patronage. It established several dispensaries which not only promoted Indian ideologies of science and medicine, but created a new image for Ayurveda in the way medicine was practiced. The first Ayurvedic dispensary was founded in 1878 by Kaviraj Chandra Kishore Sen; and as the popularity of Ayurvedic drugs increased so did the number of Ayurvedic institutions.

An obvious outcome of the revival movement that enabled Ayurveda to establish an independent professional identity lay in its success in establishing a parallel set of institutions devoted to indigenous and modern medicine throughout India. This begs the question: was the identity of Ayurveda defined by its association with Western medicine, or was it the scientific claims, which drew recognition and popularity, that justified its unique identity and professional power alongside Western medicine? The answer lies in both. The scientific and professional strengths of Ayurveda made medical encounters possible while at the same time making it available for self-criticism.

Although the revivalist movement gained a firm footing toward the end of the nineteenth century, it found expression in 1907 with the establishment of the All India Ayurvedic Congress; the Congress represented the first professional group of indigenous practitioners as the leading organization of *vaids* (practitioners of Ayurveda) in India at the time. The Congress was a voluntary association composed of individual practitioners and local provincial Ayurvedic groups that saw the reform of Ayurveda in advocating and practicing "pure" or *shuddha* school with no focus on Western modes of practice. From this evolved several regional and national associations. The princes, nobility, and the professional and educated middle classes "provided respectability and the authority to match the colonial State's support for allopathy."[26]

While efforts to frame new paradigms for Ayurveda remained paramount, some officials of the Indian Medical Service and Bengal Medical Council of Registration were threatened by the mounting pressure from the nationalists and from professional pressure from Indian medical graduates and practitioners. If nationalism is believed to be an outcome of British measures and policies in India, it also posed a constant threat and challenge to British authority and monopoly by altering the social and political climate in the country. While competition between Indian and Western medicine continued unabated, nationalism and Ayurvedic revival also became a "contested site," where ideas of a "reformed" India involved a constant engagement of political, social, cultural, and medical ideas. Several influential patrons engaged Ayurveda in their efforts to elevate the professional status; the most prominent among them was P. S. Varier, who was at the helm of the revivalist movement in the southern state of Kerala. He founded the Arya Vaidya Samajam in Kerala in 1902 with support from influential local elites and other patrons of repute. He promoted the use of efficacious drugs based in accordance with Ayurvedic principles in order to improve the practice, urging vaids to "learn to prepare medicines themselves and to maintain the standards of the drugs they used, and supply them to other practitioners or directly to patients."[27]

The first two decades of the twentieth century witnessed significant developments in the way Ayurvedic revival was conceived in relation to government policies. In 1920, the Indian National Congress supported the movement demanding state patronage for Ayurveda and passed a resolution demanding popularization of schools, colleges, and hospitals for instructions and treatment in accordance with indigenous systems of medicine and in 1921, Shyamadas Vacaspati, a reputed Ayurvedic scholar, founded a national university of Bengal, called Gaudiya Saravidyayatana, as part of the Non-Cooperation Movement.[28] An Ayurvedic wing was established in the university to protest against the introduction and spread of English style education. In the same year, Mahatma Gandhi opened the new campus of an Ayurvedic college at Delhi followed by a hospital at the Ayurvedic College in Calcutta.

It shall be noted that notwithstanding such attempts to develop indigenous medicine, the movement met with partial success. Though the movement was successful in establishing a large number of educational institutions, it was limited in setting up training courses and in creating better professional avenues for graduates in the field. Lack of uniformity in standards limited these. Nationalists and Ayurvedic revivalists disagreed on professional and educational initiatives. These conflicts led to a split between the proponents of Ayurveda which was the most serious blow to the movement—even more than the reasons which had led to its formation in the first place. Arguments between the two wings of the movement—one favoring reliance on ancient texts for promoting *shuddha* or "pure" Ayurveda and the other advocating complete integration of Indian and Western practice essentials, dislodged the goals and aspirations which nationalists had set out to achieve. Advocates of integrated curriculum recognizing that "pure" Ayurveda could not deal with the public health needs of India, led to frame a system of Ayurvedic education embodying concurrent instruction in oriental and occidental medical sciences, specifically designed to train students in the fundamental aspects of Ayurveda while simultaneously imparting knowledge of Western medical sciences. Such a concurrent teaching was envisaged as playing an important role in public health activities. But a near unanimous recognition that integration and synthesis was well nigh impossible led the proponents of "pure" Ayurveda—who were also leaders of the Ayurvedic Congress—to protest against the suggested move toward integration; instead, they demanded its immediate abolition and replacement by the *shuddha* or "pure" Ayurvedic studies. Thus, there emerged "a new type of power, invested in systems of social administration rather than lodged in individuals and titles."[29]

This was the rise of new power relations, new mechanisms of power, and new power built around medical institutions that also became contested sites within a critical sociocultural and political milieu. Differing opinions on what constituted the most efficient and scientifically acceptable paradigm of Ayurveda may have been a threat to the perceived identity of Ayurveda, coupled with the changing policies of the colonial administrators. For instance, the introduction of the Ilbert Bill in 1883 that allowed the Europeans in Bengal the right not to be tried by an Indian judge, the partition of Bengal in 1905, and the Morley-Minto Reforms resulted in several campaigns, protests, and agitation. Revivalist and nationalist concerns were increasingly linked with the intended consequences of these political moves. Thus, from the time of World War I and the Montagu-Chelmsford Reforms of 1919 that gave Indians a larger role in governing the country, Ayurvedic revival efforts were endorsed with greater authority of the advocates of Indian science and medicine.

One of the consequences of these reformational strategies was the introduction of the system of diarchy (or the system of dual power) that gave more power to provincial legislatures in the fields of health and education. Besides, the increasing entry of Indians into the legislature gave them ample grounds for nationalist voices and their demands for regeneration of Indian culture and medical knowledge. Meanwhile, the rise of the *bhadralok*, the English-educated urban Bengali bourgeoisie who remained, as Raychaudhuri[30] writes, "protagonists of the new enlightenment [the liberal and reformist movements of the nineteenth century]."

The development of an Ayurvedic college of Poona illustrates the politicization of medical revival in the postwar period, during which there were increasing problems of student unrest in Ayurvedic colleges. Led by the Civil-Disobedience or the Non-Cooperation Movement, students actively responded to the call for boycotting government schools and universities throughout India, as well as foreign goods. At Poona, political leaders founded a university after the nationalist hero, Lokamanya Tilak, where Ayurveda was taught as a major part of the medical curriculum. The second Civil-Disobedience Campaign between 1930 and 1934 witnessed even more severe events when the university was derecognized and students were imprisoned for participating in the political campaigns. As a reaction to this new policy, questions of professional claims to authority loomed large. Ayurveda was founded in 1933 by nationalist leaders in Poona in response to this perceived "threat" by colonial policies, with support from influential Ayurvedic patrons; the college gained state recognition and achieved affiliation to Poona University by 1955, later becoming a reputed and one of the best-equipped Ayurvedic colleges in the country.

Issues of engaging Unani medicine and its ideals into the Ayurveda movement were noticed at this time. Hakim Ajmal Khan, as the most influential political leader, was hailed as being the closest the Muslims had to Gandhi in terms of his political appeal. All in all, he was highly regarded by the government, respected in the Congress and among Hindus generally, and was one of the few Muslims who could feel equally at home among ulama, nawabs, and (Westernized) Aligarh graduates.[31] New rules on land ownership hurt the sentiments of the Muslim community. Evidence shows that a reputed family of *hakims* (practitioners of Unani medicine) in Kalanaur (in the northwest area of Punjab) as a family from Amritsar (also in the northern part of India), lost their *jagir* (titled land); hence, a prosperous medical school almost became extinct with only a handful of students.[32]

CONCLUDING REFLECTIONS

The national movement, so intricately linked with the revival efforts of Ayurveda, is exemplary of the manner in which issues of medical authority and dominance engage political moves to acquire legitimacy of science and medical practice. It was through these linkages that nationalism formed social and political grounds within which a progressive, scientific, and modern image of knowledge could be conceived and contested. This had a crucial impact on the colonial strategies in matters of medicine and health. Needless to say, colonial expansion was inhibited by the emerging processes of nationalist reconstruction of the past and the quest for a new identity as medico-cultural identity. Nationalism, thus, represented a political paradigm within which ideas of conflicts, disagreements, and contestations about Ayurveda could be easily expressed. Alongside this, the spur in the literary activities and literature on Ayurveda in English and the Indian vernaculars was a vehement move to "transform the hitherto relatively inaccessible knowledge into social knowledge as well as a shared system of knowledge among the practitioners."[33] This enabled the dynamic and the Western-educated Indian intelligentsia to represent an unabated "intellectual growth"[34] unparalleled elsewhere in India, and to remain at the helm in engaging Ayurveda in its "new" identity.

NOTES

1. See details in David Arnold, *The New Cambridge History of India: Science, Technology, and Medicine in Colonial India* III (5) (Cambridge: Cambridge University Press, 2000), 35.
2. Thomas S. Kuhn, *The Structure of Scientific Revolutions* (Chicago: University of Chicago Press, 1962), 7.
3. Kuhn, *The Structure of Scientific Revolutions*, 10.
4. Brahmanda Gupta, "Indigenous Medicine in Nineteenth- and Twentieth-Century Bengal." Pp. 368–78 in *Asian Medical Systems: A Comparative Study*, edited by Charles Leslie (Berkeley: University of California Press, 1976).
5. See details in Poonam Bala, *Medicine and Medical Policies in India: Social and Historical Perspectives* (Lanham, MD: Lexington Books, 2007), 72–73.
6. David Kopf, *British Orientalism and Bengal Renaissance: The Dynamics of Indian Modernization, 1773–1835* (Berkeley: University of California Press, 1969), 29.
7. "Mill's History," *Calcutta Journal* (June 20, 1819): 10–20. See details in Kopf, *British Orientalism*, 240.
8. B. T. McCully, *English Education and the Origins of Indian Nationalism* (Gloucester: Peter Smith, 1966), 254.
9. See details in McCully, *English Education*.
10. Percival Spear, *A History of India* (Middlesex: Penguin Books, 1978).
11. Bipan Chandra, A. Tripathi, and Barun De, *Freedom Struggle* (Delhi: National Book Trust, 1972), 39.
12. See details in John McLeod, *The History of India* (Westport, CT: Greenwood Press, 2003).

13. Partha Chatterjee, "The Nation and Its Women." Pp. 240–262 in *A Subaltern Studies Reader*: *1986–1995*, edited by Ranajit Guha (Minneapolis: University of Minnesota Press, 1997).

14. The destruction of traditional industries led to a progressive impoverishment of the peasants. Besides, the policy of extracting enormous land revenue further led to devastation, made worse by the meager amount peasants got in return. Expenditure on agriculture was minimal with proportionately more allocated to foreign trade and industry.

15. McCully, *English Education*, 271.

16. McCully, *English Education*.

17. John McLeod, *The History of British India* (Westport, CT: Greenwood Press, 2002), 87.

18. Paul Brass, "The Politics of Ayurvedic Education: A Case Study of Revivalism and Modernization in India." Pp. 344 in *Education and Politics in India*, edited by S. H. Rudolph and L. I. Rudolph (Oxford: Oxford University Press, 1972). See also Tanika Sarkar, *Hindu Wife, Hindu Nation*: *Community, Religion, and Cultural Nationalism* (Bloomington: Indiana University Press, 2001).

19. Michael Adas, "Contested Hegemony: The Great War and the Afro-Asian Assault on Civilizing Mission Ideology." Pp. 78–100 in *Decolonization Perspectives from Now and Then*, edited by Prasenjit Duara (Routledge: London, 2004).

20. Ian Copland, *India 1885–1947*: *The Unmaking of an Empire*, *Seminar Studies in History* (Edinburgh: Longman, 2001), 34.

21. David Arnold, *The New Cambridge History of India*, 176.

22. See Arnold, *The New Cambridge History of India*, 177.

23. Frantz Fanon, *The Wretched of the Earth*. Translated by Constance Farrington (Harmondsworth: Penguin Books, 1967), 28.

24. See details in Nick Mansfield, *Subjectivity*: *Theories of the Self from Freud to Haraway* (New York: New York University Press, 2000), 125.

25. Gayatri Chakravorty Spivak, *In Other Worlds*: *Essays in Cultural Politics* (New York: Routledge, 1987), 195–222.

26. Arnold, *The New Cambridge History of India*, 180.

27. Arnold, *The New Cambridge History of India*, 179.

28. Brahmananda Gupta, "Indigenous Medicine in Nineteenth- and Twentieth-Century Bengal," 376.

29. Nick Mansfield, *Subjectivity*, 58.

30. Tapan Raychaudhuri, *Europe Reconsidered*: *Perceptions of the West in Nineteenth-Century Bengal* (Delhi: Oxford University Press, 1998).

31. Francis Robinson, *Separatism among Muslims*: *The Politics of the United Provinces Muslims, 1860–1923* (Cambridge: Cambridge University Press, 1974), 377.

32. G. Leitner, *History of Indigenous Education in the Punjab since Annexation and in 1882* (Calcutta: Superintendent of Government Printing, 1882), 152–53. See also Roger Jeffery, *Politics of Health in India* (Berkeley: University of California Press, 1988), 46–47.

33. K. N. Panikkar, *Culture, Ideology, Hegemony*: *Intellectuals and Social Consciousness in Colonial India* (London: Anthem Press, 2002), 165–66.

34. Mel Gorman, " Introduction of Western Science into Colonial India: Role of the Calcutta Medical College," *Proceedings of the American Philosophical Society* 132, no. 3 (1988): 276–98.

Chapter Two

Teaching European Medicine in Nineteenth-Century Goa

Local and Colonial Agendas[1]

Cristiana Bastos

INTRODUCTION

The Medical School of Goa is depicted in a variety of twentieth-century sources as a Portuguese-founded institution that trained physicians who had an important role in the African and Asian colonial health services. Further research among nineteenth-century sources shows that things were not so simple and that the Medical School had a complex history that owes much to the local initiatives and to social and political engagements. In this chapter, I will argue firstly, that the Medical School of Goa was less a product of the colonial administration than an outcome of the agency of some local groups who adopted European medicine as part of a repertory of references that strengthened their own political agendas; secondly, students and graduates learned European medicine and surgery at the Medical School, but were often familiar with other healing traditions; thirdly, the Portugese administration gave little support to the Medical School of Goa throughout the nineteenth century with repeated attempts to abolish it; foruthly, the route to Africa made by some of the graduates of Goa in the nineteenth century did not correspond to programmatic decisions of the Portugese colonial administration, but to individual, familiar, and career choices; and finally, the idea of using the Medical School of Goa to raise a colonial health force was endorsed by the Portugese administration only in the beginning of the twentieth century.

TEACHING MEDICAL HISTORY IN GOA

In the mid-1940s and the 1950s, students of the Medical School of Goa were offered a course on the history of medicine in India. "India" stood for *Estado da Índia*, the Portuguese-administered Western coastal enclaves of Goa, Daman, and Diu; "medicine" stood for European medicine; and "history" stood for the tale of the pioneering actions of the Portuguese in the overseas context.

The course was created and taught by Dr. Alberto Carlos Germano da Silva Correia, popularly known as Germano Correia (1888–1967); on a second offering, it was taught by Dr. João Manuel Pacheco de Figueiredo (b. 1901). Differing less than one generation, both doctors were born in Goa, had studied at the local medical school, and had improved their training abroad. They were also self-made historians and prolific writers on a variety of topics in the humanities and the sciences. Germano Correia had a passion for physical anthropology and anthropometry. He used the racialist concepts of those disciplines for his own agenda of race and purity.[2] João Pacheco de Figueiredo combined his medical specialty in hematology and gastroenterology and a passion for research essays on Goa's medical history.[3]

Both Correia and Figueiredo regarded the creation of the Medical School of Goa as the apex of the Portuguese contribution to the development of medicine and medical teaching in India.[4] A third author, Goan doctor Pedro Joaquim Peregrino da Costa, produced an encyclopedic compilation of the deeds and actions of the graduates of Goa in the African Health Services.[5] All three of them seemed as keen about appraising Portuguese agency in the history of medicine in Goa as much as about erasing other healing practices and influences from the scenario. Why and how they did so leads us to the next sections.

HISTORY WITH AN AGENDA: GERMANO CORREIA

Born in 1888 in Panjin, Goa, Germano Correia defined himself as a "Luso-descendant." "Luso-descendants," or *descendentes*, regarded themselves as the upper crust of the local society, right next to the Portuguese viceroys and the other high ranking members of colonial governance. In the mid-nineteenth century, *descendentes* comprised less than 1 percent of the population and their influence was in decline. The large majority of the population of Goa, although baptized into Christianity with Portuguese names, was Asian; "Luso-Asians," in the words of ethnographer Lopes Mendes in his 1886 book, *A India Portuguesa*.[6]

The census of 1864 counted 555 Europeans, 2,440 descendants of Europeans, 252,203 native Christians, 127,746 "gentiles," 1,637 "moors," 356 Africans, and 197 African descendants for the *Estado da India*.[7] Not too long before, Captain Kol's 1848 figures for the same territories, organizing the data by race with a category for sub-territories and no category for religion, counted only 346 Europeans and 1,842 European descendants against 481,536 Asians, 1,096 Africans, and 516 African descendants, for the *Old Conquests*, that is, the Christianized core of Goa; in the New Conquests there were only 18 Europeans, 75 European descendants, 176,909 Asians, 38 Africans, and 21 African descendants.[8]

The minoritarian "Luso-descendants" were sometimes described as an extra caste in the dynamics of local society, whose majority was composed of groups that had converted to Catholicism in earlier generations. For the landowners, conversion had been the only way to remain on their land and keep their properties.[9] While some had fled to the outer circles and brought with them their deities and built new temples,[10] whether or not ceasing to engage in the economy of Goa,[11] many remained in the core of Goa and adopted the Portuguese ways – language, religion, diet, clothing, in sum, culture—without necessarily erasing the caste references.[12] At times, the converted Asians were the ones who perpetrated the order of the Inquisition, supported the interests of the colonizers, and enacted their very persona.[13] Differences and tensions between Goan groups in the nineteenth century were many;[14] one may highlight, however, the tension between two elite groups—the vanishing minority of "Luso-descendants" and the steadier elite of Catholic Brahmins, which contributed to the overwhelming majority of students.[15]

A strong component of Germano Correia's work is all about promoting the visibility of his own group: whether making racialist arguments about the purity of "Luso-descendants" in Asia or Africa,[16] whether writing the history of Portuguese colonization in India,[17] or in his own way of writing medical history—which was mostly about Portuguese viceroys and physicians—he set the tone for a style of narrative that was followed by João Pacheco de Figueiredo, a 1923 graduate who completed his studies at Coimbra and became the school's last director.

WRITING EUROPEAN HISTORY IN INDIA

Both Germano Correia and Pacheco de Figueiredo regarded their alma mater as the culmination of a long sequence of actions and interventions promoted by the Portuguese in India ever since the sixteenth century.[18] In their view, the very precursor of the endeavor had been the Portuguese-born physician and naturalist Garcia d'Orta (1501?–1568), who moved from Portugal to

India in 1534 as a medical assistant to the head captain, Martim Afonso de Sousa. Orta was one of the very few prominent figures of the European Renaissance with a Portuguese background. He was born to a Jewish Spanish family escaping from the Inquisition; his own move to India was probably a preventive escape from further prosecutions, something he achieved when alive—although the Inquisition still prosecuted him posthumously and symbolically burned his bones.

While in India, Garcia d'Orta had the chance to compile what became a masterpiece of the Renaissance and one of the earliest volumes of science ever printed: the *Colóquios dos simples e drogas da India*, a commented catalogue of local remedies and knowledge about the properties of plants.[19] While *Colóquios* can be interpreted today as local knowledge brought into mainstream science, or as a translation from one system of knowledge to another,[20] from Correia's and Figueiredo's perspectives Orta was the lone hero who simultaneously discovered all of these things from nature, brought civilized tools of knowledge from Europe, treated pandits and rajas, and instructed the locals on the healing arts.[21]

The next landmark in the slow path for the creation of the Medical School, after Orta's passage through India, would have been the 1687 letter from Counselor Cristovam de Sousa Coutinho to the king of Portugal asking for master physicians that could teach medicine to the local population. Coutinho argued that many lives of Portuguese subjects could be spared this way, instead of succumbing to the deadly fevers and stomach diseases that ravaged the place. To strengthen his demand, he claimed that locals were talented and prone to learning medicine and could easily provide assistance to the Portuguese, if properly trained.[22]

Germano Correia and Pacheco de Figueiredo read the document as an attempt to create an indigenous body of physicians via a Portuguese-sponsored program. The program was to be put into law in 1691 but took a long while before any action followed. Supposedly, the first response to Cristovam de Sousa Coutinho's request came from Dr. Cipriano Valadares, who taught a class in medicine at the Royal Hospital of Goa from 1702–1703.[23] Chroniclers have repeatedly referred to this "class" without offering detail regarding its contents, impact, or students. It may have never been other than what happened almost everywhere: that whoever was in the position to treat, cut, bleed, purge, and prescribe would share their knowledge and techniques with their aides and assistants and train some of them in the process. Walker argues this situation was a bed for the growth of a "hybrid medicine."[24]

The next reference to medical teaching in Correia and Figueiredo's narrative leaps to the year 1801, when António José Miranda e Almeida moved from the University of Coimbra to take the position of head physician of Estado da India and designed a new teaching curriculum for local use. The curriculum supposedly followed Coimbra's, but there is no evidence that formal teaching was ever provided on a regular basis. Most likely, the pattern of previous centuries remained: those practicing at the hospital could teach or learn from one another. Medical licenses could be obtained after ad hoc exams with the Portuguese head physician. Some of those who later helped strengthen the Medical School, such as Afonso do Rosário Dantas, achieved their credentials in this manner.[25]

Nothing suggests that the Portuguese government ever supported the initiatives of António Miranda e Almeida. On the contrary, he seemed to act on his own and without guidance from Lisbon.[26] At that time, Goa was somehow adrift from the imperial cement, purpose, or coherence, if there was one.[27] And yet, life went on in the Indian enclave, and meanings, purposes, agendas, social arrangements, and negotiations took place. Some local groups took prominence; among other things, they had an influence in the developments that led to the creation of the Medical School. But that was not what Germeno Correia was after—he was busy highlighting the Portuguese side of Goan medical history.

A DIFFERENT NARRATIVE

A critical approach to the very sources of evidence Correia and his followers used may lead us to a very different interpretation of history and suggest that the foundation of the Medical School was something other than a long series of actions the Portuguese promoted toward developing medical teaching in India. The episodes Germano Correia refers to may be better described as examples of a wider practice in the colonies: the teaching of clinical procedures during the course of actual treatment, and indeed, part of a continuum of exchanges between streams of knowledge that actually flowed both ways. European physicians in the colonies, either formally stationed there or just passing by, often shared their knowledge with their local aids in hospital and barracks. The occasional students eventually developed enough skills and status to replace their masters, a convenient thing given the scarcity of European physicians in the colonies. This sort of replacement even occurred at higher levels: historians have reported that there were indigenous head physicians in the seventeenth and eighteenth centuries.[28] Knowledge also flowed the other way around—from indigenous practitioners to their European counterparts.[29] But that fact was not worth mentioning in Correia's Lusocentric history of medicine, which jumped from a memo dated 1678 into the foundation of the Medical School in 1842, as if little existed in between—ignoring a intense flow and circulation of knowledge in bits and pieces of treatments, prescriptions, pharmaceutical compounds, practices, gestures, and acknowledgments.

THE MEDICAL SCHOOL: ITS EARLY YEARS

What was, then, the official description for the foundation of the Medical School of Goa? The authors mentioned above highlight the foundational role of Head Physician Matheus Moacho and the governor, the count of Antas.[30] However, both of them were only passing by; they had arrived recently and were about to leave. We should look somewhere else to understand what happened. There were other faculty members involved since the beginning: the Portuguese army surgeon João Frederico Teixeira Pinho; António José da Gama, the first Goan to graduate from the Medical and Surgical School of Lisbon (on a scholarship); and António Caetano do Rosário Afonso Dantas, described as a hospital physician whose only training was an informal apprenticeship at the hospital where he had entered with another sort of function.[31] More importantly, there were the students.

The first group of students of the Medical School of Goa, the cohort who graduated in 1846, included Agostinho Vicente Lourenço (later widely known for his research in chemistry), Bernardo Wolfango da Silva (whose descendants remained among distinguished Goan doctors), Felizardo Piedade Quadros, Luís Francisco Fremiot da Conceição, Pedro Gonzaga Augusto de Melo, Joaquim Lourenço de Anunciação Piedade Araújo, Francisco Xavier Lourenço, and António Luís Moreira.[32]

Students were required to be at least sixteen years old, with formal education in Latin grammar, rational and moral philosophy; they should also be able to read French—French was the language of most textbooks used in Portuguese institutions at the time. In the absence of certificates regarding previous education in those subjects, candidates could show their proficiency through ad hoc exams. Once admitted, students would go through a four-year program covering six major disciplines: in the first year, they would study anatomy, taught by the first lecturer; in the second year they would take physiology, taught by the same lecturer as anatomy, as well as Materia Medica, pharmacy and hygiene, taught by a second lecturer with the assistance of the chief pharmacist; in the third year, they would study surgical pathology, taught by a third lecturer, and internal pathology by a fourth lecturer; in the fourth year, they would take surgery and obstetrics, taught by the surgical pathology lecturer, and internal medicine, taught by the internal pathology lecturer. Their progression of knowledge was tested via regular dissertations on assorted topics, oral exams, and practical exams on patients.[33]

Students financed a portion of the school expenses. Students paid three xerafins upon enrollment, plus one xerafim for fees, and the same amount at the end of their courses. If they repeated courses they were charged twice as much; and no one could repeat a course more than once. The best student received an award of twenty xerafins. To receive their diplomas, they had to pay eighty xerafins.[34]

Further support to the school came from the budgets of other institutions—such as the Military Hospital and Health Services. The faculty was recruited from among the Health Services staff; teaching became a part of their required duties and their salaries did not burden the school's expenses. The school was to pay only "substitute lecturers" with a salary of twelve xerafins directly—but that never happened. The administration was also allocated to the faculty at no extra cost. The building belonged to the hospital and was therefore rent-free. Everything functioned with a low budget. In the early years there were hardly any teaching aids or even books. In the 1840s and 1850s more than once the head physicians ask Lisbon to send over a number of medical textbooks and other learning materials.

From then on, so say the narratives, the school became an important institution, not only for Goa, but also for the Portuguese empire: many of its graduates helped fill the chronically vacant positions of the colonial health services in Africa. After 1868, the graduates of Goa were granted, by law, two-thirds of the second tier positions in the colonial health services. That they were second tier should be emphasized, although it became conveniently erased from some of the later apologetic narratives.[35]

It is somehow remarkable that the overall account of the Medical School of Goa as a benign effect of Portuguese initiatives persisted almost intact even after the colonial era, which lasted until 1961. In spite of the expanding number of critical works examining Portuguese colonialism and local resistance,[36] the tale of the Medical School, as manufactured by Germano Correia and followers, remains largely unexamined. The reference to the pioneering character of the Medical School of Goa among its counterparts has even been incorporated into local lore: it is still possible to hear that it was "the oldest in Asia."[37] Many still share the belief that it was a great school, or at least that it produced great doctors in spite of its difficulties.[38] The extensive analysis of health and hygiene in Colonial Goa by historian Fatima Gracias restates without further examination that the Portuguese founded the teaching of medicine as early as 1842.[39] It has been taken for granted that, for better or for worse, the Portuguese administration was responsible for developing the Medical School, whether as a benevolent transfer of skills from Europe to India or as a device of colonialism to strengthen its influence. Only Meneses de Bragança, an early twentieth-century author with anticolonial positions, wrote that local efforts were the pillar of the School, which was basically ignored by the Portuguese state for several years.[40] Indeed, in the 1840s, Lisbon had little to say about what was going on in Goa. Portugal was amid political turmoil and factionalism; the government of the colonies changed rapidly and with no apparent direction. The "founding hero" of the Medical

School, Matheus Moacho, lived in Goa for a short time and returned to Portugal in 1843. Lisbon did not even acknowledge the existence of the school until 1847.[41] What comes out of the analysis, instead, is that the school was the outcome of complex negotiations between the colonial administration and local groups, whose agency was the most important element in the process.

THROUGH THE PRIMARY SOURCES: A MULTITUDE OF PRACTICES

Portuguese support for the newly founded institution was erratic and minimal. Forthcoming yearly reports from the Portuguese coordinators of the health services were filled with complaints about the lack of resources and conditions available to provide adequate teaching. In many instances, these reports also reveal that local populations held on to their own beliefs and resources regarding health and healing. Whether in a derogatory manner or in a show of curiosity about local practices and beliefs, the Portuguese officers in the colonial health services understood that their own medicine was only a part of a larger picture in which they were one option among others. There was no shortage of patients who went to the healers instead of going to the certified medical doctors. Even certified medical doctors themselves went to the healers, complained the head surgeon in 1853,[42] leaving almost no clientele to their colleagues, complained the head physician in 1856.[43] That fact brought an income problem even to the head physician: nobody ever paid for his services, as the only people who consulted him were either his own colleagues from the Medical School, the Portuguese, to whom he had the mandate of not charging, or the rare "*mestiços*" who brought in dying patients about whom the healers could no longer do anything—subject to the rule that calling a doctor in a near death situation freed the client of payment. The practice of medicine was therefore like an act of charity and hardly a lucrative job.

Whether trained in Europe or in India, physicians could not make any money from their practice in 1850s Goa. They all got jobs in the administration: of the seventy-three Medical School graduates and, together with the seventy-seven who had previously obtained their licenses directly from the head physician, all were absorbed by the state health services. On top, there was not much demand for their services, as everyone was going to healers for treatment.[44]

While the curriculum was designed beyond and against indigenous knowledge and techniques, failing to incorporate any of its aspects, students of European medicine were exposed to other sources of knowledge and healing practices. When in need they went to the healers; also, physicians and students learned from the healers. Head physicians coming from Portugal expressed dismay with what seemed a major contradiction: that Goan doctors were not only clients of local healers (*curões*), but sometimes they were the providers of traditional healing (*mezinheiros*). Also, students at the Medical School showed resistance to some of the requirements that were part of medical-surgical training, that is, anatomic dissection.[45]

Despite the formal curriculum, however, some head physicians did reveal curiosity about the potential contribution of local knowledge on the healing properties of plants. Francisco Maria da Silva Torres, who came to India in 1844 to replace Matheus Moacho, dedicated considerate energy not only to making the hospital suitable for those sensitive to caste restrictions, and also wrote vehement letters to Lisbon asking for appropriate teaching materials to improve the quality of teaching. He was also impressed by the local plants and attempted to conduct some sort of backyard clinical trial with them, using soldiers as his subjects.[46] As Garcia d'Orta had done centuries earlier, he aimed to use existing local knowledge about plants and incorporate it into mainstream medical knowledge. His efforts to promote medical teaching in Goa did not get much support from above. In 1849 he returned to Portugal and the hospital physicians and army surgeons kept the school going.[47]

José António de Oliveira, the head surgeon who assumed the interim leadership a number of times, also compiled an extensive list of books required for the proper teaching of medicine and asked the authorities in to have them shipped to India. The list included Portuguese and French works as well as a French-Portuguese dictionary. Writing in 1853, he listed many recent editions and displayed updated information about medical textbooks.[48]

Oliveira acknowledged that European-style doctors were one among several other types of health providers in Goa. Together with those who had received formal medical training, either in Goa, in Portugal, or elsewhere, there were also those who had obtained their license in the old manner, that is, directly via an examination by established doctors, either after having taken some private lessons at the hospital or through more obscure processes. Along with those, there was an undefined, albeit large, number of "gentile" doctors, in addition to village healers and illegal pharmacists who kept their herbal stores open in spite of the state regulation.[49]

Under these circumstances, some head physicians argued, one could not expect students to embrace European medicine in full. Moreover, argued Eduardo Freitas e Almeida, who took the job between 1853 and 1871, the academic background of the students was of a type that did not help the true experience of knowledge.[50]

In many cases the school seemed like a hopeless venture, with little support from Portugal; it was hardly the colonial instrument Germano Correia and followers describe. But it appears differently if we move beyond the narrative of the head physicians in charge and cease to think of it as a colonial instrument—and see it instead as a device to help create status and differentiation via educational degrees, a resource that helped them getting jobs and achieving a higher rank and prestige in a colonial society. In other words, it was in the interest of the Lusified Catholic elites—mostly the Catholic Brahmins—to have such a device for distributing titles and honors in the form of academic degrees. That did not necessarily imply the adoption of European medicine in exclusion of all others. It implied the adoption of medicine in combination with other practices, although their coexistence was not formally acknowledged.

During the mandate of João Stuart Fonseca Torrie (between 1871 and 1884), the colonial state was less and less present in the daily life of Goan health institutions. However, his reports do not exhibit the same degree of frustration as those of his predecessors—maybe due to his more realistic expectations, as he was more intertwined with Goan society and had not simply landed there from elsewhere. He nonetheless had to cope with enormous challenges, including, at times, of having to teach the entire School curriculum by himself. This fact is remembered for good and bad, both as a reminder that there had been heroes who shouldered all of the work and as evidence of the fragilities of such teaching.[51]

Portuguese support for the Medical School was verging on nothingness during Torrie's mandate. That pattern remained under his successor, Rafael Pereira, the first Goan-born director of the Medical School, trained in Goa and in Lisbon. Worse: inspections from Portugal condemned the institution and threatened to close down on grounds of low pedagogic standards. It seems clear that there was little investment in it on the part of the colonizers. We can speculate whether it would have remained as a local institution, in spite of, and eventually against, the colonial administration, serving local agendas, eventually allowing for the combination of different streams of knowledge. Rafael Pereira was himself quite sympathetic toward combining different streams of medical knowledge: during an outburst of smallpox, for instance, he argued that traditional inoculation was as good as vaccination.[52]

THE AFRICAN ROUTE

However, something occurred outside Goa that had an irreversible impact on the fate of the Medical School. The push toward empire building in Africa gave a new purpose to the school and its graduates. Joining the colonial health services in Africa had been their routine for decades. There, they could find one thing that did not abound in Goa: real jobs with real pay and real titles. Whether their training was qualified and their clinical practice was appreciated at the time is another story. Comments from some of the Portuguese sources for Mozambique regarding the Goan physicians and nurses who served there were quite derogatory.[53]

While until late in the nineteenth century, the Portuguese had not been very involved in occupying and administering the African territories they claimed to rule, since the 1880s, the mounting pressure of other European nations and the competition for influence—the "scramble for Africa"—changed everything. The remnants of the slave trade and assorted freelance enterprises were not enough to prove control over a territory; additional things were required, including military actions and the development of health services—for the troops, but also to lure and control the local populations. Eventually, Goan doctors became handy for this purpose, as some of them had already been traveling the route to Mozambique in eastern Africa.

It was precisely the "handiness" of Goan doctors for the health services in Africa that became the leading argument for the survival of the Medical School of Goa in times of adversity. Goan doctor Rafael Pereira, who headed the health services between 1884 and 1895, was probably the first who articulated the thesis in full. In his words, who, other than the Indian physicians, would be more qualified to practice medicine in Africa? Pereira used a combination of racialist and cultural arguments favoring the route from India to Africa as a way of saving European civilization. He suggested that Indian physicians were better equipped and more familiar with tropical ailments and environments than European doctors were; from that, Indian doctors should be the intermediary force between the Europeans and the Africans.[54] Rafael Pereira developed this argument at a time when the Medical School of Goa was on the verge of collapse; it had not improved from previous periods, and it still had little or no support from Portugal. It was under threat of being closed down—even though it continued to survive on its scarce resources, limited faculty, and a consistent demand from the local society, enrolling some student every year.

On his own initiative, Rafael Pereira developed the idea that the Medical School of Goa could be a tool for empire building. The Portuguese authorities, however, paid no heed to his ideas. In fact, in the following years, the prestige and shape of the school sank even lower. In 1897, the inspection conducted by the Portuguese doctor Cesar Gomes Barbosa concluded that it would better to close its doors permanently.[55]

Although Rafael Pereira had stepped down from office, his arguments prevailed. At that time, Portuguese territorial claims in Africa were challenged by Britain and Germany; as a response, the country rushed into military campaigns in Angola and Mozambique. The African colonies, which were not a popular concern until then, became a matter of national pride. Finally, in 1902, when the parliament voted whether or not to continue the Medical School of Goa, the deputy and doctor Miguel Bombarda made a speech in which he used – although he did not explicitly quote the Goan author – the very same arguments Rafael Pereira had used earlier: that the Medical School could become the ideal place to train doctors for the colonies.[56]

DOCTORS FOR THE EMPIRE

It was only then, in my understanding, that the Portuguese government truly began sponsoring the Medical School of Goa prior to which it was tolerated, but hardly supported by the central government. It served the interests of groups who valued education and praised degrees, and whose intimacy with the interests of the Portuguese corresponded to what has been depicted by postcolonial theorists as the colonial condition.[57] This interpretation of the role of the Medical School of Goa in the nineteenth century equips us to overcome the contradictions between the celebratory narrative fashioned by Germano Correia in the 1940s and the crude reports of the head physicians and surgeons Francisco Torres, Freitas e Almeida, José António de Oliveira one century before that.

In the twentieth century, due to the overall dynamics of empire building in Africa and the internal dynamics of Goan society, there was a shift in the orientation of the Medical School and Goan health services. The turning point coincides with the mandate of Miguel Caetano Dias, who, was also a Catholic but not from the higher status groups which had most profited from the existence of the Medical School. A man who had progressed in his military-medical career through personal effort and merit, Miguel Caetano Dias was a strong supporter of everything that could be modern and European about medicine. His anti-plague campaigns were conducted ferociously. His reflections on epidemics mirrored the most up-to-date understanding of infections; his medical language was permeated by military concepts.[58] His sanitary policies were the very epitome of colonial biopolitics. From then on, with the combined support of the Portuguese colonial government and local doctors, European medicine was on its way to achieving hegemony in Goan society. In the 1940s, its position was solid enough to allow the rewriting of the complex, multi-source history of medical teaching in Goa, now fashioned as an Eurocentric-Lusocentric tale, as was the one proposed by Germano Correia in his idiosyncratic history of medicine in Portuguese India.

NOTES

1. This chapter results from the project "Empires, Centers and Provinces: The Circulation of Medical Knowledge in the Nineteenth Century" (PTDC/HCT/72143/2006), funded by the Fundação para a Ciência e Tecnologia; previous research results from the projects "Medicina Tropical e Administração Colonial: Um estudo do império a partir da Escola Medico Cirurgica de Nova Goa" (PLUS / 1999 / ANT / 15157), "Medicina colonial, estruturas do império e vidas pós-coloniais em português" (POCTI/41075/ANT/2001). I am very thankful to Laurent Pordié and Harish Naraindas for their comments on early versions of the chapter.

2. Germano Correia, *Os "Luso-Descendentes" da India.* Estudo antropo-aclimológico e histórico-demográfico (Nova Goa, 1920); *Os Eurafricanos de Angola—Estudo antropológico* (Lisboa, 1925); *Os Luso-Descendentes de Angola* (Contribuição para o seu estudo Antropológico), 3° Congresso Colonial Nacional. *Actas das Sessões e Teses* (Lisboa: Sociedade de Geografia de Lisboa 1934); *Os Eurafricanos de Angola. Comunicação ao Primeiro congresso Nacional de Antropologia Colonial* (Porto: Edição da 1a. Exposição Colonial Portuguesa, 1934), I: 300–30; *A necessidade dos estudos antropológicos das populações coloniais.* Trabalhos do 1.° Congresso Nacional de Antropologia Colonial. Sep. Actas do Congresso (Porto: Ed. 1a. Exposição Colonial Portuguesa, 1934), I: 157–83; "Os Luso-Descendentes da India" *Boletim Eclesiático da Arquidiocese de Goa* II (1945–1946): 60–71, 177–85, 235–43, 283–89. See also Cristiana Bastos, "Um luso-tropicalismo às avessas: colonialismo científico, aclimação e pureza racial em Germano Correia," in *Fantasmas e Fantasias Imperiais no Imaginário Português Contemporâneo*, edited by Margarida Calafate Ribeiro and Ana Paula Ferreira (Porto: Campo das Letras, 2003), 227-53; "Race, Medicine and the Late Portuguese Empire," *Journal of Romance Studies* 5, no.1 (2005): 23–35.

3. J. M. Pacheco de Figueiredo, "Escola Médico-Cirúrgica de Goa: Esboço Histórico," *Arquivos da Escola Médico Cirúrgica de Goa*, serie A (1960) fasc 33:119–237; "Contribuição de Portugal para a Medicina no Oriente nos séculos XVI, XVII e XVIII," *Arquivos da Escola Médico Cirúrgica de Goa*, serie A (1960) fasc 33: 36–112; *A vida acidentada do Físico-mór Lima Leitão, mestre de medicina em Goa e em Lisboa* (Porto: Tipografia Sequeira, 1961.

4. Correia, *História do Ensino Médico na Índia Portuguesa* (Nova Goa: Imprensa Nacional, 1918); *História da Colonização Portuguesa na Índia* (Lisboa: Agência Geral das Colónias, 1948-58); Figueiredo, "Escola . . . " ; "Contribuição. . . . "

5. P. J. Peregrino da Costa, "Médicos da Escola de Goa nos Quadros de Saúde das Colónias (1853–1942)," *Boletim do Instituto Vasco da Gama* 57 (1943): 1–43, and 58:1–66; *Escola Médico-Cirúrgica de Goa* (*1842–1957*) (Bastorá: Rangel, 1957).

6. A. Lopes Mendes, *A Índia Portugueza* (Lisboa: Imprensa Nacional, 1886).

7. Mendes, *A Índia Portugueza*, 35–36.

8. Captain Joaquim Jose Cicilia Kol, *A Statistical Report on Portuguese India,* extracted in 1950 from official documents. Reprinted in *Selections from the Records of the Bombay Government* no. 10 (Delhi, Asian Educational Services, 1995), 328–29

9. Teotónio de Souza, *Medieval Goa*, translated as *Goa medieval* (Lisboa: Estampa, 1979. Translated in 1994). *Essays in Goan History* (Delhi: Concept, 1989).

10. Paul Axelrod and Michelle A. Fuerch, "Flight of the Deities: Hindu Resistance in Portuguese Goa," *Modern Asian Studies* 30(1996): 387–421.

11. Pratima Kamat, "Goa Indo-Portuguesa: The 'Engineering' of Goan Society through Colonial Policies of Coercion and Collaboration, 1510-1777," *Portuguese Studies Review* 9, no. 1–2 (2001): 433–65.

12. For further analysis on conversion, see Roweena Robinson, *Coversion, Conitnuity, and Change* (Sage, 1998), and Angela Barreto xavier, *A Invenção de Goa* (Lisboa: Imprensa de Ciencias Sociais, 2007).

13. Angela Barreto Xavier, "Power, religion and Violence in Sixteenth-Century Goa" *Portuguese Literary and Cultural Studies* (201) 17/18 (*Parts of Asia*) pp 25-50.

14. Rochelle Pinto, *Between Empires: Print and Politics in Goa* (Delhi: Oxford University Press, 2007).

15. Cristiana Bastos, "Medicine, Colonial Order, and Local Action in Goa," *Crossing Colonial Historiographies*, edited by A. Digby, W. Ernst, and P. Mukharji (Newcastle: Cambridge Scholars Publishing, 2010): 185–212.

16. Correia, "Os 'Luso-descendentes' da Índia"; "Os Luso descendentes de Angola"; "Os Eurafricanos de Angola."

17. Correia, *História da Colonização.*

18. Correia, Historia do Ensino Médico; O Ensino de Medicina e Cirurgia em Goa nos séculos XVII, XVIII, e XIX. História do ensino médico-cirúrgico no Hospital Real de Goa, antes da fundação da Escola Médico-Cirúrgica de Nova Goa (Bastorá: Tipografia Rangel, 1941); Figueiredo, "Escola Médico-Cirúrgica . . . "; "Contribuição. . . . "

19. Garcia de Orta, *Colóquios dos simples e drogas da India* [Goa, 1563], dir. e nota por, Conde de Ficalho, 2 vols (Lisboa: Imprensa Nacional, 1891–1895). See also C.R. Boxer, *Two Pioneers of Tropical Medicine: Garcia d'Orta and Nicolás Monardes* (London: Wellcome Historical Medical Library, 1963). M. N. Pearson, "First Contacts between Indian and European Medical Systems: Goa in the Sixteenth Century," in *Warm Climates and Western Medicine*, edited by David Arnold (Amsterdam: Rodopi, 1996), 20–41. Mark Harrison, "Medicine and Orientalism: Perspectives on Europe's Encounter with Indian Medical Systems," in *Health, Medicine, and Empire: Perspectives on Colonial India*, edited by Biswamoy Pati and Mark Harrison (Delhi: Orient Longman, 2006), 37–87.

20. Richard Grove, "Indigenous Knowledge and the Significance of South-West India for Portuguese and Dutch Constructions of Tropical Nature," *Modern Asian Studies* 30 (1996) 121–43.

21. Correia "O Ensino"; Figueiredo "Escola."

22. Figueiredo, "Escola. "

23. Germano Correia, "Os percursores do ensino da medicina e cirurgia em Goa," *Arquivos da Escola Médico-Cirúrgica de Goa*, série A, fasc 20 (1947): 38–67; Figueiredo, "Escola," 121.

24. Timothy Walker, "Remedies from the Carreira da Índia: Asian Influences on Portuguese Medicine during the Age of Enlightenment" *The Portuguese Studies Review* 9 (2003): 1–21

25. Bastos "Medicine, Colonial Order," 203.

26. Fatima Gracias, *Health and Hygiene in Colonial Goa* (*1510–1961*) (New Delhi: Concept Publishing House, 1994). Bastos, "Medicine, Colonial Order."

27. As Patrick Wilden explored in *Empire Adrift* (2005), somehow resonant of Saramago's "Stone raft," the trope "adrift" appropriately depicts some of the moments of the Portuguese colonial venture. Sadly, there is little analysis of nineteenth-century Goa, except for E. Carreira, "Índia," in *Nova História da Expansão Portuguesa. O Império Africano, 1825–1890*, vol. 10, edited by V. Alexandre e J. Dias (1998) and the recent Rochelle Pinto, *Between Empires*, as well as the older ethnographic works of Lopes-Mendes, *A Índia Portugueeza* (1886) and Bragança Pereira, *Etnmografia da India Portuguesa* (1921). That absence is most remarkable since the nineteenth century is of the utmost importance for understanding imperial power. For the history of Portuguese colonialism, nineteenth-century Goa may provide enough evidence for an original interpretation of the nature of relations between centers and colonies, between the rulers, the ruled, and the in-between. From our own projects, some articles have been putting out preliminary analyses: Bastos "Doctors for the Empire: The Medical School of Goa and its Narratives," *Identities* 8, no.4 (2001): 517–48; "The Inverted Mirror: Dreams of Imperial Glory and Tales of Sub-alternity from the Medical School of Goa," Etnográfica VI, no.1 (2002):59–76; "Um Luso Tropicalismo"; "O Ensino"; "Race, Medicine"; "Medical Hybridisms and Social Boundaries: Aspects of Portuguese Colonialism in Africa and India in the Nineteenth Century," *Journal of Southern African Studies* 33 (2007): 767–82; "Borrowing," "Medicine, etc"; R. Roque "Sementes contra a varíola: Joaquim Vás e a tradução científica das pevides de bananeira brava em Goa, Índia (1894–1930)," *História, Ciências, Saúde -Manguinhos* 11 (2004): 183–222; M Saavedra, "Percursos da vacina na Índia portuguesa—séculos XIX e XX," *História, Ciências, Saúde-Manguinhos* 11 (2004): 165–82

28. Pearson "First Contacts" (1996); Walker "Remedies"; Bastos "Medical Hybridisms."

29. Along the same lines of interpretation, Walker "Remedies" has documented the interactions between European and Indian medical systems up to the eighteenth century. Ines Zupanov—"Drugs, Health, Bodies, and Souls in the Tropics: Medical Experiments in Sixteenth-Century Portuguese India," *The Indian Economic and Social History Review* 39 (2002)—analyzes how healing was embedded in the practices of the different social actors. Further evidence about the families of those who became the first formal students at the Medical School of Goa suggests that there was some overlapping between local medical knowledge and the institutional medical teaching that the Portuguese reportedly promoted. The older Peregrino da Costa, who graduated in 1850, is depicted as a good clinician and a master of the local *segredos* (literally "secrets" for botanical remedies) by his own descendant, later a chronicler of the Medical School. The younger doctor describes the older one as "a clinician of great reputation, who also used indigenous medical plants that, according to the mindset at the time, were so-called 'secrets,' and one who, by genial clinical intuition, was the first to prescribe a salt-less regimen for edema and hydric retention, cardiac or renal, fifty years before the works of Widal; a clinician who, due to the faith of the people in his therapeutics, was admired throughout the boroughs of Goa" (Costa *Escola*, p. 28).

30. Costa, *Escola*, 14.

31. Bastos, "Medicine, Colonial Order."

32. Costa, *Escola*.

33. Francisco Maria da Silva Torres (Fisico-mór do Estado), José António d'Oliveira, (Cirurgião-mór do Estado), and António José da Gama, *Regulamento para a Escola Médica de Goa*, ms, Nova Gôa, 18-8-1845, AHU, s 12, m. 1987.

34. Silva Torres, d'Oliveira, and da Gama, *Regulamento*, 12.

35. Costa, *Escola*.

36. Axelrod and Fuerchs, "The Flight"; Souza, *Medieval Goa*; Pratima Kamat, *Farar far Crossfire: Local Resistance to Colonial Hegemony in Goa*, 1510–1912 (Panaji: Institute Meneses de Bragança, 1999).

37. Bastos, "Doctors"; "Inverted."

38. Recently collected internet clippings confirm it; in a posting to the article "Goa's pathetic public health system," where Dr. Nadkumar Kamat deprecates the public health institutions of Goa (Dr. *Navhind Times,* 7 April 2003), an anonymous author argues that the lamentable state of things nowadays contrasts what had been a matter of excellence for Goa's former medical school hospital, which had been founded by the Portuguese and was the oldest in Asia. www.colaco.net/1/nanduGoa'sPatheticPublicHealthSystem.htm, accessed on 11/11/2003. Even more recent clippings re-state the belief: abemdanacao.blogs.sapo.pt/266857.html, accessed September 9, 2008.

39. Fatima Gracias, "Quality of Life in Colonial Goa: Its Hygienic Expression," in *Essays in Goan History*, edited by T. Souza (Delhi: Concept Publishers,1989): 185–203.

40. Menezes Bragança, "A Educação e Ensino," *Índia Portuguesa* 2 (1923):145. The day may come when the founding of the Medical School may be celebrated as a local act and in a way, evidence that the Portuguese did not entirely rule Goan agendas. The Medical School of Jakarta, founded in 1857 by the Dutch colonial rulers, is today celebrated as a breeding ground for nationalism, for the roots of the nationalist movement began there. See Lisbeth Hesselink, "Crossing Colonial and Medical Boundaries: Plural Medicine in Java 1850–1910," *Crossing Colonial Historiographies*, edited by A. Digby, W. Ernst, and P. Mukharji (Newcastle, Cambridge Scholars Publishing, 2010): 115–41.

41. Bastos "Doctors"; "Inverted Mirror."

42. José António d' Oliveira, *Relatório do Estado das Repartições de Saúde do estado da Índia* (11/7/1853), AHU, s12, m1987.

43. Eduardo de Freitas e Almeida, *Oficio* de 8-2-1856 AHU, s 12, m 1987

44. Almeida, *Oficio*, 12.

45. Almeida, *Oficio*, 12.

46. Francisco Maria da Silva Torres, *Oficio* de 21-4-1846, AHU, s12, m 1987.

47. C. Bastos, " O Ensino"; "Corpos, climas, ares e lugares: autores e anónimos nas ciências da colonização," *A Circulação do Conhecimento: Medicina, Redes e Impérios*, edited by C. Bastos and R. Barreto (Lisboa: Imprensa de Ciências Sociais, 2011): 25–58.

48. José António d' Oliveira, *Relatório do Estado das Repartições de Saúde do estado da Índia* (11/7/1853), AHU, s12, m1987.

49. Oliveira, *Relatório*, 12.

50. See Eduardo de Freitas e Almeida, *Oficio* de 11-7-1854; *Oficio* de 8-2-1856 *Oficio* de 4/6/1861. See also Bastos, "O Ensino."

51. It deserved a satirical portrayal in the famous chronicles "Farpas" by Portuguese nineteenth-century writer Ramalho Ortigão, as quoted by Peregrino da Costa (*Escola*, 22–23) and became a sort of a legend and inside joke for the Medical School.

52. Rafael António Pereira, *Relatorio do Serviço de Saúde, Referido aos Annos de 1897–99, 2a. Parte Epidemia de Variola*; *Ataque Infecioso*; *Defeza Organica e Immunidades* (Bastorá, Goa: Rangel, 1900). Bastos, "Borrowing, Adapting, and Learning the Practices of Smallpox: Notes from Colonial Goa," *Bulletin of the History of Medicine* 83 (2009): 140–62.

53. In 1893, the Portuguese doctor José Serrão de Azevedo, while heading the health services of Mozambique and supervising a number of physicians who had graduated in Goa, produced very negative comments about the quality of their training. He acknowledged that while the Portuguese schools could not guarantee the excellence of every one of its graduates, the School of Goa produced "extraordinary specimens," which, in his view, indicated that their school was not up to the level of what a medical school should be (*Relatorio do serviço de saude da província de Moçambique 1893*, Arquivo Histórico Ultramarino, Serviço de Saúde do Ultramar, maço 2817). He further argued that the impossibility of practicing in Portugal as evidence of that poor quality; but the fact that they were allowed to practice in Africa created a double standard situation. In his opinion, the school should either be improved or shut down. For further discussion see Bastos, "Race"; "Medical Hybridisms."

54. Rafael António Pereira, *Relatório do Seriço de saúde da Índia* (30 October 1889). AHU, rm 12, no. 1988.

55. César Gomes Barbosa, *Relatório da Inspecção ao Serviço de Saúde do Estado da Índia, 1897*, AHU, s12, m1988,

56. Miguel Bombarda, "A Escola de Nova Goa," *A Medicina Contemporanea—hebdomanario portuguez de sciencias médicas*. Série II- tomo V, XX, no.12 (1902): 93–95.

57. Homi Bhabha, "Of Mimicry and Man," (28 October 1984):125–33.

58. Miguel Caetano Dias, "Relatorio do Serviço de Saude, Referido ao anno de 1902," *Arquivo Historico Ultramarino*. For a discussion see Bastos "Germ Theories in a Colonial Setting: Medical Theories and Military Practices in a Late Nineteenth-Century Goa, India" *EASST Review* 17, no. 4 (1998): 9–12.

Chapter Three

Ayurvedic Pharmaceuticals

Contesting Economic Hegemony

Madhulika Banerjee

India has been home to a number of diverse systems of medicine for a long period of time, all of which are known to have coexisted *sans* major conflicts, be it the medical encounter between Ayurveda and Unani systems of medicine (the latter came with the Sufis and the Turks) or medical exchange after the codification of medical knowledge. However, the colonial encounter was like none before as the colonizers were self-conscious carriers of the fundamental transformations of European society, polity, and economy through modernity. Modern science, the greatest emblem of modern European society, combined with the strength of the capitalist enterprise and economy, was fully backed by the power of the modern institutions of governance. While all of these may have been in their formative stages in the nineteenth century, the colonial power posited these as a powerful contrast to those existing in India. For the first time in Indian history, thus, was a hostile encounter that significantly transformed and, sometimes diminished, its own culture, economy, and politics like none before. There was no dialogue and absorption that had characterized encounters between cultures, especially those of systems of knowledge before. This was particularly true for the Indian systems of Medicine—Ayurveda, Unani, and Siddha, as also a host of "local health traditions" (not textually grounded, but in people's memories and practices).

HUMORAL ENCOUNTERS

The encounter of Ayurveda with biomedicine under British colonialism was preceded by the system of medicine practiced in Britain between the sixteenth and eighteenth centuries. Western medical knowledge, in its early years, was based on body humors. Thus, when European physicians first encountered Indian medicine they found a system that was, in its broad outlines, completely recognizable.[1] Like the European system, Ayurveda presented a theoretical underpinning of humoralism, coupled with a similar attitude to the use of plant medicines, and indeed many exact parallels in diagnosis and therapy.[2] While some scholars[3] have highlighted the differences in the practices of the two, others have remarked that except for Zimmerman,[4] who has attempted a comparative casting between the Ayurvedic corpus and the Hippocratic/Galenic corpus, we do not have a comparative rendering of an Indian and European medical theory in the eighteenth century: the moment of its contemporary meeting.[5] Naraindass has done comparative rendering in his analysis of a well-known text of the time, J. Z. Holwell's *An Account of the Manner of Inoculating for the Smallpox in the East Indies*[6] in which he argues that

> Holwell sets out not merely to describe the practice of inoculating for the smallpox, as the title of the essay seems to suggest, but to record a theory and practice of its origin, cause and therapeutics.

He also highlights the fact that "there is none of the anguish of translatability that comes from any felt notion of incommensurability."[7] Also, there is an elaborate presentation of the "cool regimen" and its creation and maintenance which is necessary for preventing of smallpox, together with the practice of inoculation. These are all derived from the classical texts, but are practiced by trained vaids as well as other specialists. Interestingly, neither Ayurveda nor Unani had any effective remedy for smallpox, as Habib candidly explains.[8]

The above analysis is relevant here for several reasons. First, while it must be acknowledged that the case of Howell cannot be generalized to reflect the complete interaction between the British and Indian medical knowledge, it does illustrate a different encounter that ensures continuity in its character which Pearson saw as an informal "dialogue" between Western and Indian practitioners.[9] Second, this study falsifies the claim of most historical literature that there is not much theoretical underpinning of the humoral system that could have credibly travelled from India to Britain. Third, an explanation of exchange of knowledge indicated credulity of Indian medical methods by British doctors, which contrasts with later methods discovered in Britain and enforced by the colonial authorities in India, particularly with respect to smallpox. Differences in understanding this disease and its management signified the character of contestation over the larger parameters of medicine and health between the colonial government and its subjects—these differences were articulated over a period of time.

THREE STAGES

The colonial encounter took place in three stages, all of which were responsible for the irrevocable transformation of Ayurveda in the modern period. In this context, Arnold suggested that

> the relationship between Western and Indian medicine, needs to be looked at in more pluralistic and dialectal terms, terms that allow for a continuing interaction between the two during the long history of colonial rule in India, or that express the relationship as a protracted epistemological struggle which says more about the nature of political and economic power under colonial rule, than about the abstract merits of two, contrasting, competing, but not wholly incompatible medical systems.[10]

The three stages in the medical policy of the British colonial regime toward indigenous medicine have been discussed at length by Bala.[11] The first phase coincides with the consolidation and expansion of the colonial rule from the late eighteenth until the middle of the nineteenth century with a concomitant increase in the establishment of medical institutions. There are substantial numbers of records of European doctors, botanists, and pharmacologists, listing the flora, fauna, and other natural and medical resources of India which were used to understand the newly emerging categories of diseases in biomedicine. Besides, Whitelaw Ainslie's *Materia Medica of Hindoostan* (1813) and Sir William Jones's *Botanical Observations on Select Indian Plants between 1790–1800*,[12] added to the growing appreciation for indigenous knowledge.

The establishment of cantonments and hospitals necessitated an encounter with the local systems of medicine, thus calling for official recognition and inclusion into newly created institutions. The founding of the Native Medical Institution in 1822, followed by the Calcutta Sanskrit College and the Calcutta Madrasa, where parallel instructions were carried out in indigenous and translated medical texts, through the vernacular medium, proved it all. Although these were to train natives in medicine for the expanding empire, it implied that appreciation of Ayurveda and Unani was to be combined with their recognition as compatible when taught along with the new medical sciences of Britain and Europe.

At the same time, indigenous drugs deserved merit for economic reasons by the government. A historical survey of the standardization of crude drugs has shown that the different methods used to control the quality of these substances had developed alongside the increase in knowledge of the characters, properties, and constituents of the plants and drugs involved.[13] At the same time, the comparative costs of European and "native" medicines in favor of the latter, provoked the Medical Stores Department to urge their usage. This led to two important developments—the publication of O'Shaughnessey's *Bengal Pharmacopoeia*,[14] the first compendium dealing exclusively with the properties and uses of medicinal plants used in Bengal in 1837, and the establishment of a medical laboratory by the governor-general of India in council for preparing medicines to study their effects. This initiated a drug-substitution policy of European drugs by indigenous drugs, which meant that the supply of European medicines could be limited to just those medicines for which no native drug could be used.[15] Thereafter, several indigenous drugs were added to the *British Pharmacopoeia* and introduced in government dispensaries, visibly following the cholera epidemic of 1839–1840.[16] But this was not encouraged beyond a point when it affected the market for imported plant materials because of the belief that new purification and standardization procedures were perfected in Britain, which, coupled with advances in chemistry and their application to pharmacology, made the imported plant materials superior to Indian drugs. Since instituting these changes was a formidable task, the best option was to import them in the long run. Thus, George Wyatt, writing in the preface to K. L. Dey's monograph on *Indigenous Drugs of India*, lamented

> the few that are good are neglected and largely so, because the cry for imported drugs and European pharmacy is obliterating all knowledge in the time ecumenical experience of the useful drugs of this country.[17]

Thus, while expenditures on imported plant materials increased very rapidly, the Medical Stores Department often declared that indigenous drugs ought to be used more generally and the ones available in a crude and uncouth form be given laboratory treatment before administration. This set off a debate on "drug-substitution" that was to continue for a long time, signifying a disagreement within the government on this policy, albeit with a minority supporting Indian drugs. This also formed the basis for the Drug Enquiry Committees of 1895, 1930, and in later years. The committees did not alter colonial policies but their terms of analysis have long-term implications for Ayurvedic drugs in the future, as discussed in the following sections.

This is the beginning of the two strands that dominate Orientalism—the most benevolent perspective of the Western mind on Indian medical systems. One was to accord the systems of knowledge a parity of status with that of

Western medicine, by combining the best in the two forms of medicine for training the new generation of British doctors. The other was the recognition of indigenous drugs and significant formulations in the *Ayurvedic Pharmacopeia*. Both had implications for the way Ayurveda was shaped under colonial rule as well as in later years.

The second phase of the development of Ayurveda under colonialism is identified with the beginning of the controversy between Orientalists and Anglicists in the early nineteenth century, which changed British attitudes toward all forms of knowledge in India. Macaulay's famous Minute on education in 1835 provided the basis of this controversy, and new grounds for higher education which, as Brass sees them, became and has always remained in Western knowledge of all kinds, a power game that served the fundamental aim of constructing the superiority of their knowledge system.[18] By creating a section of people trained in this system, this superiority was inducted into the consciousness of an elite (and it would have to be the English-educated elite), ensuring its hegemonic position as no form of coercion possibly could.

The influence of the political developments and the concomitant changes in the British medical profession did have their echoes in India, as seen in the Medical Registration Act of 1853 and the formation of the General Medical Council about the same time. The latter raised issues on the policy of the colonial state as regards the hakims and vaids, practitioners of Unani and Ayurveda, respectively. In the 1880s, however, the government of India decided against introducing registration of the Western-style doctors on the grounds that they were not strong enough to combat the outcry which the hakims and vaids would raise.[19]

There are several ways of interpreting this phase of the encounter. One interpretation is that there has been a heavy reliance on the decisions on medical education—that in 1822, establishing the Native Medical Institution in Calcutta, and its abolition in 1835 which transformed it into a body more akin to a British medical college of the time. Accordingly, it is clear that both the symbolic support to the indigenous systems offered by the first institution, and the symbolic threat embodied in the change to the second, were less significant than has been argued. The former was, by most accounts, of no sign of a serious commitment by the Orientalists to the cause of the resuscitation of the indigenous systems, nor did the second decision mean that state support was denied to indigenous practitioners.[20] Yet another way of looking at it is that this contestation left a positive legacy which had long-term consequences. Although the Orientalists lost the debate on educational policy in British India, they provided an ideological platform for an indigenous movement that has transformed medical learning in modern South Asia. The leaders of this movement adopted technology, ideas, and institutional forms from the evolving cosmopolitan system to found pharmaceutical companies, colleges, and professional associations and to reinterpret traditional knowledge.[21] A third way of understanding this perspective is to perceive the Orientalist-Anglicist controversy as the overarching logic that subsumed an empirical reality of vibrant diversity. The traditional systems continued to be the point of health reference for a majority of the people of the colonial state, while these systems were in a state of ferment and anxiety about what they clearly saw was a challenge to their legitimacy. The response of the systems was articulated slowly and came to fruition only in what will be seen to be the third phase of colonial policy and the encounter.

The third phase can be located from around 1890, when the colonial government was strong in terms of territorial acquisition and legal supremacy. More significantly, from the 1880s, the practice of medicine under the empire became a history of techniques and policies—of education, epidemiology, and quarantine—the discovery of pathogens and vectors and the segregation of races. Dominant in colonial medicine was tropical medicine; from the late 1870s, tropical medicine—its ideology European, its instrument the microscope, its epistemology the germ theory of disease—served the interests of the dominant economic groups and obscured the relationship of disease to social structure.[22] The power of this orientation has also been variously interpreted, primarily in terms of its significance in the consolidation of the colonial state in general. While its role in the larger power structure is not of relevance here, what is important is that the support provided by the colonial state to this perspective on health, disease, and medicine came to exert an increasingly powerful hold over the bodies and minds of the Indian people, to the extent that it fashioned their thoughts, feelings, and desires and made them come to think of India in medical terms, like a diseased body politic that required the services of an expert physician.[23] This meant that the biomedical perspective of complete disdain for the traditional systems was consolidated during this phase. So what had been slowly building up from around the 1830s, now found a clear articulation in a typical relationship which had three dimensions: first, the biomedical tradition never fully conceded the possibility of any traditional system being thoroughly competent and comprehensive in itself; second, it sought to assess the efficacy of traditional medicine, with the understanding that the only acceptable way to do this is by modern scientific methods; and third, that a pharmacopoeia along the lines of British, or any other well-known "format," is essential for its authenticity. As a result, Ayurveda and Unani were seen as "unscientific" and, thus, obsolete forms of medical knowledge that needed to be discarded. Jeffery argues, though, that the government had conflicting policies being proposed and supported on the issue of indigenous systems and their practitioners. While on the one hand, there were those who opened indigenous medical colleges, there were others who argued that the improvement of the training of hakims and vaids was a part of the policy of the government because they were recognized as the real source of medical care and attention for the majority of the populace for a long time to come.[24] This development went alongside major events in Britain at the time including a rejection of the humoral basis of medical practice and the triumph of clinical medicine.

IMPLICATIONS FOR AYURVEDA

From this stage of the encounter onward, therefore, the survival of Ayurveda, Unani, and the others was entirely dependent upon innovations and their creative responses against the powerful colonial machinery clearly pitted against them. Evidence shows that they were no passive recipients of colonial power. Groups and associations of hakims and vaids formed by this time to understand the implication of colonial policies. When many petitions and exhortations for their medical and scientific value failed to elicit any substantial response and invited ridicule instead, they had to explore alternative avenues of expression for the purpose—and this was provided by the market.

The growth of modern markets, in general, and the market for medicines in India, in particular, are important markers of this stage of the encounter. As discussed earlier, concern about importing crude and finished drugs into India remained paramount. Kumar, however, demonstrates how this profitable venture—in which India was the largest market of all manufacturing countries for finished products of the chemical industry by World War I—was unlikely to change.[25] In all instances of modern industry development, the state was an active proponent, enabling them to settle in their gestation period before being able to make a profit. In this sense, a major factor was lacking as far as Ayurveda and Unani drugs were concerned. Yet, other kinds of changes and shifts were occurring, more toward the end of the nineteenth century. The growth of the middle class—not merely the educated, English-speaking elite—formed the backbone of the nationalist movement at this time, and also the increasingly successful small traders, large landowners, and emerging industrialists. Jeffery[26] argues that this is what made the broad-based market gain prominence, helping the breakdown of old oligarchic patronage that made the indigenous practitioners successful until this time. Thus, there were changing market opportunities and the profession responded to them. It is in this frame that we can see new directions—the development of the Ayurvedic Pharmaceutical, the proliferation of the modern textbooks of Ayurveda, and the creation of the Ayurvedic clinic, each recasting the old in new recognizable forms—of the pharmaceutics, the *Samhitas* and physician-teacher tools. Leslie points out that the Orientalists paved the way for Ayurveda to adopt from biomedicine, but how they did so is even more interesting. Parts of the codified texts of Ayurveda that dealt with physiology and anatomy were recast in a form that was then dominant and, therefore, legitimate. This set the stage for new writings by Indian practitioners of Ayurveda, renowned among which were Ray's *History of Hindu Chemistry*, Seal's *The Positive Sciences of the Ancient Hindus*, and Murti's *Fundamental Principles of Ayurveda.*[27] These and several others projected the changing image of Ayurveda, thus demonstrating that the practitioners of Ayurveda and the elite medical men, created a space for themselves and learned how to zealously guard as well as grow in it—to create a modern space for themselves, so as to remain in contention for some locus of power. Prakash offers a lucid viewpoint on this. He adds,

> To think of science's authority in India and the modern Indian elite as products of a translation between the lines is to bring another history into view—a history of an irreducibly different Indian modernity forged in the interstitial spaces opened by the process of translation. Viewed as a process of translation, the elite does not appear as a copy of the original, but as a ghostly double that resists identification as a copy by asserting difference. This is a history that sits oddly beside not the heady celebration of modernity as progress and its stinging denunciation as the colonisation of the mind, and reveals the emergence of the indigenous elite's counter-hegemonic aspirations in the translations of Western modernity.[28]

While this portrait could be largely concurred with, some qualifications about the Ayurveda elite, however, need to be made. Even in their assertion of difference, aspects of "colonization of the mind" were reflected in their desire to follow, and not challenge, the scientific parameters laid down by the colonizers. This becomes clear as we look at one of the most powerful counter-hegemonic arguments that went on to become an all-time classic. Stated thus:

> Whatever new sophistication the West dangles before us as the latest necessity for any socially or scientifically mature society, ancient India has already produced it. Worn of its shine by now, it continues to be pathetically paraded, reflective perhaps of the grave paucity of either imagination or enterprise of what is no longer elite in Indian society. [29]

The character of the new medicines, of their ready availability and immediate effects, and also the economy of producing them on a mass scale, provided new initiatives for manufacturing new drugs. This was also conveyed in the Orientalist approach of de-linking the drugs from the system of diagnosis and treatment, as evident in the first and second stages of the encounter. It is important to note that the development of the modern pharmaceutical itself followed an almost independent trajectory in Europe, combining developments in science with developments of capitalist production systems. It seemed as though the pharmaceuticalization process was the inevitable link of modern medical knowledge systems to the momentous developments of economy and society. Hence, the birth of the Ayurvedic pharmaceutical was inevitable, if Ayurveda were to find a place in the rapid socioeconomic changes at the time, also effectively posing an alternative to biomedicine in India.

If the Orientalists had their inheritors, so did the Anglicists. For the latter, the future of modern India lay with institutionalization of biomedicine and the rejection of all nonscientific modes of medical knowledge. Their idea found congruence with nationalists who envisioned a free India aspiring to have all the features of modernity. This congruence created a powerful lobby of nationalists which conflicted with other developing political interests. The grey areas in this conflict between the two kinds of nationalists that resulted in the contestations around Ayurveda within a larger debate on the terms of discourse of nationalism cannot be dismissed. These will be discussed in the section on nationalist contestations, following our discussion on the founding moment.

Unusual as it may seem, this turns out to be a classic case of the confrontation between two systems of knowledge in which traditional knowledge enjoyed legitimacy at one level but was forced to come to terms with a constructed ideology of the rational supremacy of the other and incorporate changes within its own form and content.[30] The confrontation between the Ayurvedic and biomedicine manifests this, and also the resolution. Ayurveda began as modernity's Other, given its stark difference and supposed epistemic and ontological differences with biomedicine as it was evolving over a period of time. But under colonial rule, the system tried to cast itself in the mirror image of modernity. What emerged from this effort was a double, mimicking many of the features, but never quite making it to the real thing. Modernity's Other could also have charted an alternate course of modernity and provided another interpretation, another trajectory of the modern. This is examined in the last section.

BIRTH OF THE AYURVEDIC PHARMACEUTICAL

The late nineteenth century is the founding moment for the protagonist of this chapter—the Ayurvedic pharmaceutical. A rough country-wide mapping of firms at this time illustrates that the manufacture of Ayurvedic drugs was established in different parts of the country—in Bombay (Dhoot Papeshwar, 1888), in Kerala (Arya Vaidya Sala Kottakkal, 1901), Coimbatore (Arya Vaidya Pharmacy, 1902) and in the heart of the empire, in Calcutta (Kalpataru Ayurvedic Works, 1884) and Dhaka (Shadhona Aushadhalaya, 1888). They were set up by practicing vaids, who first evolved methods by which these medicines could be mass produced for the market. The way in which these firms produced, packaged, and marketed their medicines, learning new methods in each of these areas from the newly established pharmaceutical industry in Europe and the United States, transformed Ayurveda in ways they would not have envisaged. This was a technological transformation effected to make an ancient system provide the knowledge base for a new "product." Significantly, this response offered by vaids straddled the two spheres in which modernity was hegemonic—in epistemology and the market. It was a move away from any reliance on influencing colonial state policy on medicine which put practitioners in competition with their Western counterpart, including state-sponsored and private practitioners. Well-known vaids took initiatives to prepare medicines on a larger scale than they had done before, fixed price lists, and published advertisements alongside setting up educational institutions whereby they could perpetuate the teaching of and training in Ayurveda. But the inability to cope with the growing market, however, became apparent in Ayurveda. This made large-scale production absolutely necessary, a requirement that was taken up by *kaviraj*-entrepreneurs to build a large number of successful Ayurvedic firms. It meant that the premises, number of people employed, and the amount produced increased in size. More importantly, it meant that new procedures for manufacturing medicines would be the same as traditional ones, which retained the six forms in which Ayurvedic medicines were made—*bhasmas*, *churnas*, *lehas*, *arishtas*, *asavas*, and tablets. In 1884, however, a company called Kalpataru Ayurvedic Works established by Gananath Sen aimed to produce Ayurvedic medicines on a large scale for sale at moderate prices, preparing them with the aid of modern machinery in the form of pills, tablets, and powders.[31] This is the first indication of the change in the form of medicines as a result of a change in the production process. What it did for Ayurveda was to make the medicines easily available, off the shelf and for a price, removing the earlier linkage with the physician, and endowing the patient with a range of choices in the market. This development caused controversies and conflicting interests. The change in the form had far-reaching implications for Ayurvedic practice. While vaids who were practicing for a long time, objected to the new move, the latter gained popularity with the rise of teaching hospitals and colleges. Conflicts ensued because of the recognition that the older practice of the healer preparing medicines for his patients was not merely "small-scale" production, but a form with a particular healer-patient relationship in diagnosis and treatment.[32] Thus, when the production system needed to be changed, practitioners saw it as symptomatic of a shift in the perception of the efficacy of Ayurvedic medicine as not well equipped to handle acute situations and as an attempt to redefine parameters of treatment in order to follow the hegemonic ideology of Western medicine; this meant that the illness structures were modified to conform to Western ideas in identifying illness as disease. While this fulfilled the marketing requirement, for Ayurveda already had medicines for illnesses that biomedicine claimed to be creating anew, it also created new choices for the large clientele, thus laying the foundation of the Ayurvedic pharmaceutical industry in India. The context of *standardization* of Ayurvedic medicines was, however, not set at the time of large-scale manufacture. As early as 1866, Ayurvedic drugs were being examined not only in isolation from the system of knowledge of which they were a part, but were subjected to "laboratory treatment before administration"[33] in government dispensaries and hospitals. The pressure of these tests and standardization procedures, however, was not confined to deriving economic benefits, but the developing knowledge in biomedicine offered a pharmaceutics challenging the fundamentals of the older forms of drugs, which meant that the criteria for efficacy and validity were to be transformed accordingly. Testing the drugs for efficacy that produced varying results for Ayurvedic and Western drugs raised new doubts about their authenticity. This marked the beginning of an ongoing debate that is still continuing.

Most of the drug companies were concentrated in Bengal. Gupta interprets the popularity of Ayurvedic drugs in terms of the Ayurvedic Renaissance that was part of the Bengal Renaissance, which served a nationalist purpose of extending medical relief through Ayurvedic medicine to the rural population. This is not without merit, though it seems more likely that the immediate material gain must have been an important consideration for a new production decision. However, when viewed in the context of developments in critical reflection and thought in the profession, manifest in new textbooks and "histories"of Ayurveda, the latter reveals a reflective response of a system of thought to a more powerful, dominating one.[34]

The Bengal Renaissance was followed closely by a significant political development of the *swadeshi* (of one's own country) movement. An important strategy of the movement was to substitute colonial products with those produced at home and a boycott of foreign goods. In the early years of the twentieth century, there was a popular recognition that colonialism had adverse effects on the Indian economy and that any opposition to colonial rule must include an opposition to its economic policies and structure. In response, the movement also set up new Ayurvedic medicine manufacturing concerns to provide further boost to the emerging Ayurvedic pharmaceutical concerns.

The Ayurvedic pharmaceutical industry has not provoked the imagination of economists' writing on colonial India. The analysis offered here is an attempt to sketch an outline by correlating the political ideologies of the time with the dominant ideology of production for which our argument is based on the existing literature on industrial development of the period[35] as well as a comprehensive article on the overall pharmaceutical industry in India during the colonial period.[36] During the *swadeshi* period, small firms played a pioneering role, especially in Bengal where professional Bengalis opened new units of industry in the days of patriotic fervor following the partition of Bengal in 1905.[37] Goswami sees this development as a response to the slogans of economic nationalism of Jagdish Chandra Bose and Prafulla Chandra Ray.[38] While economic nationalism and reassertions of the significance of Ayurvedic medicines in the market may have enabled the growth of pharmaceutical industries, the foundation of a similar firm in Kerala is a case in point. P. S. Varier, a vaid of a distinguished heritage of physicians, founded the Arya Vaidya Sala in Kottakkal in 1901, believing that Western medicines appear more attractive to people because they were palatable, gave quick relief, and came without dietary restrictions. With the modifications he suggested in the manufacture of drugs also ensuring a longer shelf-life and quicker transportation to a wider market, Varier's pharmaceutical company prospered significantly.

Besides, other firms continued to produce Ayurvedic medicines in their original forms but with a modified production process using new technologies. These are best understood if located in the larger context of emergence of new chemical and pharmaceutical manufacturing firms in India in the early decades of the twentieth century—for instance, Alembic in Parel (Bombay) and Baroda[39] and the legendary Bengal Chemical and Pharmaceutical Works in Calcutta. The latter was set up by the strident technocratic nationalist P. C. Ray, whose company was already successful in making the latest chemical formulations for Western medicine. He pioneered the production of modern chemical formulations based on the active principles of the components of the compound drugs of Ayurveda with a belief that a fresh appreciation of the knowledge of pharmacology in Ayurveda would appear credible and be acknowledged only if combined with a form of modern chemistry of Western medicine. This provided yet another dimension to the negotiation of the identity of Ayurvedic medicines. Both had long-term effects in the manufacture and consequent identity of Ayurvedic medicines with their own inheritors of late twentieth-century formulations in the Indian market.

Enthused by Ray, the Calcutta Chemical Company was set up with new technology to manufacture soap, toothpaste, and herbal cosmetics, thus catering to the new middle-class public and the new market for goods of mass consumption. This development owed its existence to two Bengali families, the Mitras and the Dasguptas, whose ideas of technocratic nationalism meant aligning the Indian capital with the latest technology in the world market; they had brought the latest techniques in soap and cosmetic manufacture from England, the United States, and Germany.[40] For Ayurvedic manufacturers, this meant a significant positioning of their products, for Ayurvedic formulations could then be recast into newer forms of products. An entire range of products, free of the disturbing issues of validation on scientific lines of the efficacy and standardization of Ayurveda, could then be produced with the guaranteed response from the embedded consumer. This provided yet another avenue for modern Ayurveda, one that holds well today.

World War I served as a turning point for the growing drug industry in India. It reduced imports, stimulated industrialization by import substitution, disorganized the supply lines of the expatriate firms, and brought increased liquid assets into the hands of the bazaar speculators and traders for investment in the industrial field.[41] This explains how professional men, including Ayurvedic practitioners, were able to garner capital resources which also came from their own profits or from progressive landlords willing to risk a part of their income from land for patronizing industrial development.[42] In the inter-war period, as Ray suggests, while small firms continued to play an important role in industries which could be run without large capital, small firms like Dabur switched to the manufacture of allopathic medicines because they were more profitable to make, while the Ayurvedic medicines were difficult to sustain economically. Yet, the inter-war period was a time of increased conflicts between foreign capital and indigenous enterprise. The two constraints identified in economic research on long-term industrial growth in India—the limited size of the market and backward technology—were absent at this time and Dabur did well in the inter-war years.[43] The situation, however, changed after the war when multinational corporations discovered this market as well as the limitations of the indigenous industry. They chose products that were the lifeblood of *swadeshi* firms.[44] While many firms were able to sustain themselves even until the 1930s, the hold of the multinational corporations had become strong. Thus, lack of capital and the low level of technology led to the marginalization of indigenous industry generally. Ray and Goswami indicate that these enterprises did not survive beyond the 1930s for a variety of reasons, though principally, for a lack of capital and business experience.

While the lack of capital could have been due to their own shortcomings in fund management, the problem with technology arose because of the inordinate costs of the new technology available in Europe and the United States. In the entire literature on economic history, this is bemoaned and the several factors which built up this situation are identified in "deindustrialization" and "discriminating protection." Two issues need serious consideration here. As Kumar indicates, in the industrial evolution of Ayurvedic and Unani drugs, strategic protection or the "forced protection" of the War period had absolutely no role to play in the promotion of these drugs but owed their expansion to individual entrepreneurship, the support of admirers, and the quality of their products.[45] This was one Indian industry that built on its own initiative and remained innovative throughout in response to competition. Yet, it is seen as not innovative enough. It took as given, the frame of production and distribution of medicines embodied in large-scale production, mechanization and marketing, from the colonial and European experience. Fascinated by the achievements of the Industrial Revolution, it was never envisaged that a completely different approach to the rationale of products, capital, markets, and consumers could have produced a different kind of technology altogether. This rationale, if created by combining past experiences of industrialization in India or, indeed, the long history of the making and distribution of medicines with the transformations taking place in the society and economy in the nineteenth century, had greater chances of being *swadeshi*. It could also have been a product of the culture of the medical system of Ayurveda, as its technique and market. I argue that this would have had a greater potential for *swaraj*, whereby a different structure of market and capital might have emerged instead of the movement from colonialism to neo-colonialism, that is, from the European managing houses to the multinational corporations. But it is well known that the process of industrialization and economic development followed the dominant ideology of production and exchange in the modern world, and that the modern capitalist forces of production were considered the "forward" march of technology, while all else was "backward" and so, the logic of development in India could not have been very different.

Ayurvedic medicine firms were on the margins of industrial development until after independence in 1947 when they slowly took advantage of the new provisions in legislation and the changing character of the market. With the development of indigenous heavy capital industry, in machinery and chemicals, they established themselves as part of the development of the pharmaceutical industry as a whole. The pattern of development, however, continued to be in terms of using more modern machinery and increasing standardization, which meant that the terms of discourse on technological development remained the same. The hegemonic ideology that was set by the contestations around Ayurveda and the structures of production that emerged in the colonial economy led specifically to the twin processes of commercialization and standardization of Ayurvedic medicines. The details of these processes embodied the larger complexities of economy and polity as they developed through postcolonial policies of industrialization with emphasis on science and technology.

NATIONALIST CONTESTATIONS AND AYURVEDIC PHARMACEUTICALS

The emergence of the Ayurvedic pharmaceutical and the rising nationalism were parallel responses to the changing political climate in the country. Practitioners with either entrepreneurial or political acumen were at the helm of both responses and commanded authority primarily on the basis of their knowledge of Ayurveda. As entrepreneurs, they contributed to their political standing and, at the same time, provided a new forum for the emerging voices of the community. The first organized response to British policies from the Ayurvedic community was the formation of the All India Ayurveda Mahasammelan in 1907. Its members were directly embroiled in a controversy with the government over the policy to register doctors trained in the biomedical system by the Medical Registration Act passed in the various provinces in 1910. By this time, colonial administration with its altered structure of legality and jurisprudence (in which administrative classification alone gave legitimacy to the existence of institutions or groups) exclusively recognized doctors trained in Western medicine. The new legitimate political forum for Indians, the Indian National Congress, came under increasing pressure from this lobby. As early as 1893, resolutions urged to raise a scientific medical profession in India by throwing open fields for medical and scientific work to the best talent available and indigenous talent in particular.[46] The first Congress resolution that specifically complained about the way indigenous medicine was denigrated by laymen or antagonists, without allowing the practitioners to present their own case, was passed in 1918.[47] The resolutions from 1920 onward demanded government patronage for Ayurveda. Under pressure, the provincial governments began to grant assistance to Sanskrit *Mahavidyalayas* imparting instruction in Ayurveda, to help in establishing new Ayurvedic institutions. Several provincial governments passed acts of legislation through the Boards of Medicine regulating indigenous practitioners and establishing government institutions.[48] This was a departure from earlier practice, but the overall attitude of the central authorities remained the same with continued support to Western medicine and bypassing the interests of indigenous practitioners, as evident from the Indian Medical Association formed in 1928. The association was formed under pressure from the General Medical Council in Britain and had close links with the Congress and leading doctors trained in Western medicine who were also important leaders in the party. But the contestations around Ayurveda cannot be understood merely from the point of the different kinds of moves and counter-moves made by the practitioners on the basis of the support among the congressmen and political leaders. For this was the time when nationalism, as an ideology, governed not only the anticolonial movement but also articulated a vision of future India. This included the terms in which the larger philosophy of the relationship of modernity with tradition of a postcolonial vision of India was to be set, with emphasis on the role of modern science and technology. The most important among these were the long-term implications for society and politics and the positions on science and technology. Nandy provides a framework for a second colonization, a colonialism that "colonizes minds in addition to bodies and releases forces within the colonized societies to alter their cultural priorities once and for all."[49] Those in the realm of the second colonization were not homogenous—they were the inheritors of both the Orientalist and Anglicist schools of the colonizers—that is, the traditionalists and the neo-traditionalits or modernists, respectively. The contestations between them were conducted within broader colonial perspectives, as discussed below.

Gandhi provided a new position that differed on the basic parameters of analysis from the other two. The traditionalists and neo-traditionalists believed in the relevance of Ayurveda for modern India in the same way as the Orientalists did for most knowledge systems of the Orient, constructing a unique identity of Ayurveda. Besides, in defense of the Ayurvedic knowledge, the traditionalists believed that the innate value of Ayurveda would be available in the modern period if the traditional structures of learning and practice were continued. The neo-traditionalists, on the other hand, believed that the hostility to Ayurveda could be allayed by "translating" its precepts into categories and concepts understood by modern science. This process could establish close links between the two medical systems. This would also ensure the survival of Ayurvedic heritage. The manufacturing concerns and educational institutions embodied beliefs of modern medicine resulting in a syncretism between Ayurveda and Western medicine.[50] They also provided a the base for the controversies on teaching and learning, the *shuddha* (pure) versus integrated Ayurveda controversy that continues even after independence. While there was a confrontation on these questions in epistemology, in the parameters of the market, both *shuddha* (made according to traditional formulae) and integrated (adapted from the pharmacology to make new medicines) products coexisted without debate. The industrial production structures and methods for Ayurvedic medicines and the coexistence of *shuddha* and integrated Ayurveda illustrate the poverty of the nationalist discourses by even those who were at the helm of the defense for Ayurveda.

Contrasted with the above two were the inheritors of the Anglicists, the modernists who were in the mainstream of Indian politics. The modernists believed in the wonders of new medicine and technology that Indians had to learn from Europe. With the unfolding of discoveries in chemistry and physiology, aggressively marketed by new methods devised by the pharmaceutical industry in Europe, the generations of doctors trained in the medical colleges set up by the colonial government eagerly awaited their transmission to India. This provided a new model for a health service structure, as evident in the recommendations of the National Planning Committee (1938). The Committee was Nehru's brainchild and was inspired by Soviet planning models that drew a blueprint for post-independent India. Its report demonstrated a significant epidemiological orientation with a significant suggestion of a "health worker" for the rural areas, who would not be an imposition from the outside, but one who belonged to the local area and would be trained to deal with local health requirements. However, as Jeffrey states, the committee dealt delicately with the issue of indigenous medicine, suggesting that young vaids or hakims might make good health workers, with additional scientific training. The report attacked some of the features of indigenous practice, such as their unwillingness to divulge the contents of some of their remedies and also proposed an Indian Pharmacopoeia which would investigate the effectiveness of traditional remedies.[51]

To sum up, the perpetuity and survival of Ayurveda was facilitated by the establishment of the Ayurvedic Pharmaceutical in the nineteenth century, which signified standardization and homogenization of both form and procedure of manufacture. It also necessitated the transformation of the Ayurvedic texts and practice into a single body of knowledge. A critical assessment of colonial policy shows that this encounter and the role of the colonial state both led to the transformation of Ayurveda. Yet, it may be argued that given its scientific base of reason and knowledge, the triumph of biomedicine was inevitable. It might appear that state support for Western medicine must have been forthcoming because of the recognized innate superiority and its ability to demonstrate cures extended by the pharmaceuticalization of medical knowledge and the professionalization of practice. However, historical research bears no evidence to this.

A reappraisal in historiography would be useful here to understand the experiences of Britain and India in terms of the development of the pharmaceutical industry in Britain. In nineteenth-century Britain, conflicts between the old orders of apothecaries and small-time medicine makers and the new pharmaceutical houses was being articulated and resolved. Two types of medicine could be identified with the two groups: patent and rational. This, however, did not reflect the actual state of affairs of therapeutics at the time. Rational therapeutics, based on a scientific understanding of the mechanisms of action of effective drugs was a long way into the future.[52] Two important issues were of concern here: adulteration and how it was to be combated, and false claims of the efficacy of these drugs and how that was to be dealt with. Both of these had implications for legislating the manufacture of medicines and claims for their efficacy and standards.

Two important scientific developments in synthetic chemistry and in biology profoundly influenced the creation and growth of the pharmaceutical industry and related research. Both these developments were taking place in other countries of Europe, particularly Germany and France. While the flourishing German chemical industry created synthetic chemical treatments with disease-specific treatments, the application of Pasteur's germ theory revolutionized ideas about therapeutics by developing antitoxins against specific diseases.[53] It is in this context that the experience of Henry Wellcome and his certification as a chemist, based on his laboratories of testing and standardization in the late nineteenth century, is very illustrative. His company, which had set up its own laboratories for research and had come up with its own antitoxins around 1894, was clearly embarked upon reaping the obvious commercial potential of such an enterprise. Just at this time his plans nearly ran aground because extending the research in this direction of testing necessitated animal, testing which required a registration under the 1876 Cruelty to Animals Act. No commercial establishment had hitherto been thus registered, as this was the prerogative of laboratories in institutions of learning. The Pharmaceutical Society strongly opposed his claims on the basis that his was a commercial enterprise and could never satisfy the rigorous norms of science, reflecting the desire of the pharmacists to ally them closer to the medical profession than the marketplace. This was because the market was identified with chemists and druggists, who suffered a dubious reputation, as discussed before. As Wellcome could have shifted his business outside of Britain, the issue became ultimately a choice between losing a very profitable commercial institution and agreeing to the registration. The signal to the entire industry, then, was that it would be profitable in the long run to move away from the unfettered claims and systems of production toward a more "scientific" orientation.

INDIAN CONTRAST

Clearly, then, the encounter of biomedicine with Ayurveda had a very different substance and, therefore, could not admit of the same historical trajectory. Two points of comparison between Britain and India in the nineteenth century can emerge from the above account. First, that in epistemic terms, Ayurveda was radically different and incompatible with biomedicine. Its early difference would not have looked so significant to the British, much like in the eighteenth and early half of the nineteenth century when Ayurveda's affinity to the humoral tradition of Britain was obvious. Later, when the antagonisms between biomedicine and herbal medicine in Britain itself became sharp, with the increasing power of the "scientific" medicine in Britain in the second half of the nineteenth century, Ayurveda's response was provided principally by its very strong living textual tradition. In this resource, the herbal tradition was weak and, therefore, its erasure was far more fundamental in Britain than in India. Thus biomedicine emerged partly out of the creation of a new paradigm of body and illness, but also through the displacement of older structures of the practice of medicine, as has been described above. In this, the state had to mediate between contending parts of the civil society that claimed legitimacy either by newer epistemological or commercial forms.

The second issue is that of the development of the market and its relationship to the state. The strong links between the commercial and professional interests of the chemist and druggists, overtaking the initial (early nineteenth-century) significance of the apothecaries and forging of a new relationship with the doctors, helped establish the modern pharmaceutical industry in Britain. In other words, it was an organic development of a new industry impelled by the forces of power and medical culture emanating from within the society. In India, however, the market for the new medical products was created by the colonial state itself—by the direct altering of the rules and regulations for its own administration and officials—and also by legitimizing through endowed grants and support to the new medical colleges and the new perspective on healthcare, which had a clear negating effect on the Indian systems of medicine. The initial, substantive resistance to this came from the market and later from the political organizations of Ayurvedic medical practitioners, which also became part of their necessary legitimizing process of being accepted in the framework of a modern society.

Gandhi's visions of "science" were first outlined in the *Hind Swaraj*[54] (1909) and subsequent writings until his death in 1948. The overall impression that pervades both in social science and active politics is that he was "anti-science" and recommended a retrograde vision for the future of India with his talk of "*gram swaraj*" and "*ram rajya*." As an acknowledged leader of the Congress from 1919 onward, this was one issue on which he had no sympathy from his followers and even admirers, including Nehru. Gandhi raised several points of contestation about Ayurveda, hardly any of which were identified by anyone else at the time.[55] More importantly, Ayurveda did not exhibit a spirit of inquiry and humility to the unknown, similar to that of modern science. The tenor of Gandhi's criticisms about the inability of Ayurveda to keep abreast of modern research (and incorporating it into its practice) seems dangerously close to the modernist and British criticism of it. I would argue that the aggressive self-confidence of Ayurveda, with respect to all new knowledge, is rooted in its claim of the basics, the parameters of analysis in the *panchamahabhutas* (the principle of five elements of which the human body is made of) and some others, rather than everything that needs to be known about health and medicine. Thus, there is a need to understand even the "confident" responses of vaids, to check what appears to be representative of Ayurvedic knowledge.

Thus, in the contestations of colonial authority, these myriad forms were acquired by a significant body of practitioners of Ayurveda. They cast themselves into different forms that they believed would make them appear more legitimate for the state, as well as for projecting a future vision of modern India visualized through these forms. The survival of the latter under colonial rule was evident by the early twentieth century and, hence, the strategies undertaken ensured their long-term survival, marked by a continued debate over these issues.

NOTES

1. M. N. Pearson, "The Thin Edge of the Wedge: Medical Relativities as a Paradigm of Early Modern Indian-European Relations," *Modern Asian Studies* 29, no.1 (1995): 141–70.
2. D. Wujastyk, *The Roots of Ayurveda* (New Delhi: Penguin, 1998), 35.
3. D. Kumar, *Disease and Medicine in India: An Historical Overview* (New Delhi: Tulika, 2001), xvi.
4. F. Zimmerman, "Gentle Purge: The Flower Power of Ayurveda." Pp. 209–23 in *Paths to Asian Medical Knowledge*, edited by C. Leslie and A. Young (Berkeley: University of California Press, 1992).
5. H. Naraindass, "Of Therapeutics and Prophylactics: The Exegesis of an Eighteenth-Century Tract on Smallpox." Pp. 95 in *Disease and Medicine in India: A Historical Overview*, edited by D. Kumar (New Delhi: Tulika, 2001).
6. J. Z. Holwell, "An Account of the Manner of Inoculating for the Smallpox in the East Indies" (1767). Pp. 195–218 in *Indian Science and Technology in the Eighteenth Century: Some Contemporary British Accounts*, edited by Dharampal (Delhi: Impex India, 1987).
7. Naraindass, "Of Therapeutics and Prophylactics," 96–97.
8. I. Habib, "Inside and Outside the Systems: Change and Innovation in Medical and Surgical Practice." Pp. 75 in *Disease and Medicine in India: A Historical Overview*, edited by D. Kumar (New Delhi: Tulika, 2001).
9. M. N. Pearson
10. D. Arnold, *Colonising the Body: State Medicine and Epidemic Disease in the Nineteenth Century* (Delhi: Oxford University Press, 1993), 286.
11. See details in P. Bala, *Imperialism and Medicine in Bengal: A Socio-historical Perspective* (New Delhi: Sage, 1991).
12. Bala, *Imperialism and Medicine in Bengal*, 41.
13. Bala, *Imperialism and Medicine in Bengal,* 50.
14. Bala, *Imperialism and Medicine in Bengal*, 48–49.
15. Bala, *Imperialism and Medicine in Bengal*, 51.
16. Bala, *Imperialism and Medicine in Bengal*, 48–49.
17. George Wyatt, cited in in K. L. Dey, *Indigenous Drugs of India* (Calcutta: Thacker, Spink, 1896), ix.
18. Paul Brass, "The Politics of Ayurvedic Education: A Case Study of Revivalism and Modernization in India." Pp. 342–71 in *Education and Politics in India*, edited by S. H. Rudolph and L. I. Rudolph (Cambridge, MA: Harvard University Press, 1972).
19. R. Jeffery, "Doctors and Congress: The Role of Medical Men and Medical Politics in Indian Nationalism." Pp. 62 in *Education and Politics in India,* edited by M. Shepperdson and C. Simmonds (Aldershot: Avebury, 1988).
20. Jeffery, "Doctors and Congress," 62.
21. Jeffery, "Doctors and Congress," 62.
22. C. Leslie and A. Young, eds. *Paths to Asian Medical Knowledge* (Berkeley: University of California Press, 1992), 179.
23. R. Macleod and M. Lewis, eds. *Disease,Medicine and Empire: Perspectives on Western Medicine and the Expercience of European Expansion* (London: Routledge,1988), 7.
24. Jeffery, "Doctors and Congress," 65.
25. Anil Kumar, *Medicine and the Raj* (New Delhi: Oxford University Press, 2001), 361.
26. Jeffery, "Doctors and Congress," 62.

27. P. C. Ray, *A Complete History of Hindu Chemistry from the Earliest Times to the Middle of the Sixteenth Century* (Calcutta: The Bengal Chemical and Pharmaceutical Works Ltd., 1903). See also B. N. Seal, *The Positive Science of the Ancient Hindus* (Delhi: Motilalal Banarsidass Publishers Pvt Ltd., 1915).

28. G. Prakash, *Another Reason: Science and the Imagination of Modern India* (Princeton: Princeton University Press, 1999), 51–52.

29. L. Cohen, "The Epistemological Carnival: Meditations on Disciplinary Intentionality and Ayurveda" in *Knowledge and the Scholarly Medical Traditions*, edited by Don Bates (Cambridge: Cambridge University Press), 320-43.

30. Owing to the efforts by historians of science, following Thomas Kuhn's *The Structure of Scientific Revolutions*, it is readily accepted now that a confrontation between two or more knowledge systems is never a purely "logical" or "rational" affair. Fundamentally different knowledge systems, or what Kuhn calls "paradigms," involve different understanding of what it means to be logical or rational. Disputes between such fundamentally different knowledge systems can never be resolved empirically, for they involve different ideas of what constitutes "hard core" evidence and how to go about testing the validity of a "fact." Therefore, a paradigmatic confrontation—say, between Aristotelian physics and the Newtonian physics—is always resolved "externally," that is to say, factors other than the pure or intrinsic merit of the argument finally decide the matter. It could be the need of the society concerned or its power equation, among other things.

31. B. Gupta, "Indigenous Medicine in Nineteeth- and Twentieth-Century Bengal," in *Asian Medical Systems: A Comparative Study*, edited by C. Leslie (Berkeley: University of California Press, 1976), 368-82.

32. This is discussed in some detail in M. Banerjee, *Power,Knowledge, Medicine: Ayurvedic Pharmaceuticals at Home and in the World* (Hyderabad: Orient Blackswan, 2009).

33. *Proceedings of the Government of India*, July–December 1866. Quoted in Bala, *Imperialism and Medicine in Bengal*, 51.

34. A textual analysis of these alone can be used to demonstrate the same hypothesis, but remains to be done.

35. O. Goswami, "Sahibs, Babus and Banias: Changes in Industrial Control in Eastern India 1918–1950," in *Entrepreneurship and Industry in India 1800–1947,* edited by R. K. Ray (New Delhi: Oxford University Press, 1992). See also A. K. Bagchi, *Private Investment in India 1900–1939* (London: Cambridge University Press, 1982).

36. D. Kumar, *Disease and Medicine in India: An Historical Overview* (New Delhi: Tulika, 2001).

37. Rajat Ray, ed. *Entrepreneurship and Industry in India: 1800–1947* (Delhi: Oxford University Press, 1992), 259.

38. Goswami, "Sahibs, Babus and Banias," 249.

39. D. Kumar, *Disease and Medicine in India: An Historical Overview* (New Delhi: Tulika, 2001), 371.

40. Ray, *Enterpreneurship and Industry*, 250.

41. Ray, *Entrepreneurship and Industry*, 50.

42. Ray, *Entrepreneurship and Industry*, 259.

43. A. K. Bagchi, *Private Investment in India, 1900–1939* (Cambridge: Cambridge University Press, 1972). See also Ray, *Entrepreneurship and Industry.*

44. Goswami, "Sahibs, Babus and Banias," 252.

45. A. Kumar, *Medicine and the Raj*, 382.

46. Jeffery, "Doctors and Congress," 161.

47. Jeffery, "Doctors and Congress," 167.

48. P. Brass, "The Politics of Ayurvedic Education," 345–46.

49. A. Nandy, *The Intimate Enemy: Loss and Recovery of the Self under Colonialism* (Delhi: Oxford University Press, 1983), xi.

50. C. Leslie and A. Young, eds. *Paths to Asian Medical Knowledge* (Berkeley: University of California Press, 1992), 177–208.

51. Jeffrey, "Doctors and Congress," 170.

52. R. Porter, "Before the Fringe: 'Quackery' and the Eighteenth-Century Medical Market," in *Studies in the History of Alternative Medicine,* edited by R. Cooter (Oxford: Macmillan Press, 1988), 2.

53. E. M. Tansey, "Pills, Profits, and Propriety: The Early Pharmaceutical Industry in Britain," *Pharmaceutical Historian* 25, no. 4 (1995): 3–8.

54. *Hind Swaraj* (Ahmedabad: Navjivan Press, 1909).

55. J. P. S. Uberoi, *Science and Culture* (New Delhi: Longman, 1977); See also A. Nandy and S. Visvanathan, "Modern Medicine and its Non-Medicine Critics: A Study in Discourse" in *Dominating Knowledge: Development, Culture, and Resistance*, edited by S. A. Marglin and F. A. Marglin (Oxford: Clarendon Press,1990), 145-84; S. Sahasrabuddhe, *Science and Politics: Essays in Gandhian Perspective* (New Delhi: Ashish Publishing House, 1991); and S. Visvanathan, *A Carnival for Science: Essays in Science, Technology, and Development* (New Delhi: Oxford University Press, 1997). In the spate of writings that came in the wake of the *Hind Swaraj* centenary celebrations, there was an increased focus on ideas of *satyagraha* and nonviolence, rather than on technology, with the exception of *Knowledge Swaraj: An Indian Manifesto on Science and Technology* (Hyderabad: Knowledge in Civil Society, 2010).

Chapter Four

Corporal Contestations

A Fragmentary History[1] of British Indian Medical Improvement, 1836–1913

Shrimoy Roy Chaudhury

In the year 1913, on an auspicious day in the Hindu calendar, a group of esteemed gentlemen of the British Presidency of Bengal gathered in Chinsura, Hooghly, to inaugurate a charitable dispensary.[2] Following the performance of Hindu religious rituals to mark this occasion, Jogendralall Chowdhury took the stage to remember his father, the benefactor of the charitable dispensary, the late Badan Chandra Chowdhury. The charitable dispensary was formally opened by the Raja of Burdwan, the proprietor of one of the biggest zamindaris in Bengal. Effusive words poured forth in memory of Badan Chandra Chowdhury, the first native Sub Assistant Surgeon of the Hooghly Imambara Hospital, and a disciple of James Esdaile, who had introduced mesmerism for surgical operations on patients at a time when chloroform was yet to be discovered.[3] In 1855, on receiving a transfer order to the North West Provinces, he resigned from his post in the Hooghly Imambara Hospital to take up private practice, which proved much more lucrative. He drew a substantial clientele from among the Bengali professional class and the landed elite of Hooghly and Burdwan districts. Son of an employee in the Calcutta General Post Office who was burdened by a huge family, Badan Chowdhury came to amass a fortune, having himself become the proprietor of a substantial zamindari. He bequeathed the first property he had bought in Chinsura to the cause of founding a charitable dispensary and "charities which formed the ancestral Dev Sheba or worship of family gods."[4]

Held in the quadrangle sharing the threshold of the house, a religious ceremony preceded the actual inauguration of the charitable dispensary. Thereafter, amid a profusion of bunting and flag hoisting in the street front, the formal inauguration started with the head Brahmin Pundit Mahamohopadhyay Shib Chandra Sarvabhouma of Bhatpara[5] garlanding the Maharaja of Burdwan as an act of "benediction" in "oriental style." This was followed by notes of address by the delegates.[6]

Read from the vantage point of the post *swadeshi* movement political milieu of Bengal, the inaugural ceremony represents the emergence of *daktari* as a vernacular idiom of articulating concerns about national health. This chapter aims at studying the pre-history of *daktari*, the vernacular word for identifying modern medical practice introduced by the colonial state, from this vantage point. This is not to claim a moment preceding *daktari* as much as a study to understand the conditions of possibility for *daktari* to emerge as a vernacular idiom of therapeutic agency. I shall explore this question in four registers—firstly, the investigative frame within which W. W. Hunter put forward his questions about the legitimacy of the appropriation of the Hooghly Imambara Endowment—the existing "covenant" with the Shias; secondly, the framing of Haji Mohamed Mohsin's will; thirdly, the significance of the establishment of the Hooghly Imambara Hospital in the British pursuit of legitimacy through the Hospital; and finally, the emergence of *daktari* as a site of political contestation over claims to speak for the body as an imagined realm of governance on the occasion of the inauguration of the late Badan Chowdhury's charitable dispensary. Hence it is also a study of the embeddedness of that imagination in the shifting ideas and practices of corporality exemplified by the colonial rulers.

THE HOOGHLY IMAMBARA ENDOWMENT: A CASE OF "MISAPPROPRIATION"

Writing in 1872, W. W. Hunter would argue that it was the covenant between the ex-king of Awadh, the late Wajid Ali Shah and the British state, exhibiting the former's faith in British rule and pledging to recognize the interests of the Christians and Muslims as one, which had prevented the Shia community from siding with the "Puritan" rebellion of the Wahabis.[7] He argued that this was so, despite the fact that the British government had neglected the interests of the community by "misappropriating" funds endowed for religious piety by Haji Mohamed Mohsin to be used for establishing and running an English College. He claimed that in pursuance of *takiyah*, or "Law of the

Pious Fraud," the Shia community had stood fast beside British rule against Wahabi invitations to join their cause even as they pretended to dissimulate sectarian differences with the Wahabis for the greater good.[8]

Hunter's analogy between *takiyah* and the Law of the Pious Fraud is significant. *Takiyah* or *taqiya* was a practical principle which relieved the Shia subject from the obligation to hold on to the beliefs of faith in a generally hostile environment. It was not merely allowed, it was itself an obligatory duty, attributed to the Imams, including Ali.[9] However, unlike *taqiya*, acts amounting to simulation or dissimulation of one's identity was treated by modern Western jurisprudence as a morally contested terrain; the figure of the Pious Fraud emerged through the subject's confession of the act while defending himself or herself in the court of law as a juridically responsible agent, or otherwise, through the attribution of particular actions as characteristic of the Pious Fraud by historians. The attribute of intentional ignorance, which distinguished the Pious Fraud, implicated the latter of misappropriating his or her authority to deceive the other, with the intention of doing well to the other.[10] To that extent, the "Law of Pious Fraud" could measure up to a wise act, but it was, no doubt, always a subject of litigation, where the subject could be found guilty of harming broader interests in favor of pursuing self-interest. It was precisely this connotation which led Edward Gibbon, at the end of the eighteenth century, to distinguish the real miracle workers, the African Holy Confessors, from the African Catholic "Pious Frauds"—the latter having shown impunity to "compose fictions" and ascribe their "polemical works" to the most venerable names of Christian antiquity. The source of the contest between the Arians and the Trinitarians, which Gibbon contextualized in the hostile world of the fifth century inhabited by religious and barbaric forces, was the African Catholic Church and the frauds it committed in the names of the venerable Christians to fight off the barbarians.[11]

Hunter's equivalence between *taqiya* and the law of the Pious Fraud, therefore, was an act of productive misrecognition. No doubt, by positing the covenant with the late Wajid Ali Shah as the fundamental reference for assessing the feelings of the Shia community toward the British government, Hunter discovered the covenant to be the source behind what he felt to be a formidable bond between the British state and the Shias in India. Hunter's assumption of the certainty offered by the connection between the directive part of Hunter's referred covenant and its predictable part which was meant to ensure that the direction was carried out in certain specific ways, was precisely what was not available in *taqiya.* The translation reflected Hunter's own sense of anxiety around the realization that the Indian Mussalmans, though bound by their own law to live peaceably under British rule, continued to question British rule, often in a "fanatical" manner. On perusing the judicial testimonies, Hunter found out that many Wahabis operational in and around Delhi were actually peasants of Eastern Bengal, forcing him to understand through a litigious engagement how the Wahabis managed to procure sympathy from their coreligionists for a cause which they did not deserve to by the law of Sharia.

Hunter's anxiety about restoring the proper object of the "covenant" was not unwarranted. After all, how could one discount the fact that Wajid Ali Shah had been "pleased" to be part of the covenant while living as an exiled émigré in Metiabruz, Calcutta, at the pleasure of the British government as its pensioner, after Lord Dalhousie, legislating in the voice of a doctrinaire against mis-governance, had him ousted from Awadh. Adding poignancy to the irony of Hunter's claim of a covenant with the Shias was the fact that while in exile Wajid Ali Shah had composed a memoir, which was translated from Persian as "Sorrows of Akhtar: An Autobiographical Account of the Deposition and Imprisonment of Sultan-i-Alam Wajid Ali Shah, the Last King of Oudh." This covenant, Hunter revealed, had been selectively circulated in the form of pamphlets among the Sunnis and the Wahabis in ways that would hit like "darts" and rankle the hearts of "their Wahabi and their Sunni countrymen" to no ends, leaving his late Majesty's Wajid Ali Shah's party's loyalty shining with "redoubled luster."[12] No doubt much was invested in the idea of the covenant.

Paradoxical as it may sound, the prefiguration of the Shias as the Pious Fraud was symptomatic of the anxiety around the fact that the covenant itself was a sham device, which had been enabled to represent the scale on which the behavior of the Shia would be measured. The idea of the covenant with the Shias was a productive means of intervening, assessing, and asserting British influence against the grain of Wahabi movements across the Gangetic plain. In that the covenant resembled the sham devices used in placebo trials in the nineteenth century, on which was acted out the drama of intentional ignorance, where both the experimenter and the patient subject were expected to be unaware of each other's ulterior purpose at least partially.[13] At an elementary level, in the nineteenth century, these placebo trials involved the use of blindfolding the patient to prevent the visual sensations from affecting the results of the psychic patient's investigation. The blindfold, it was expected, would enable the body to speak for itself in its essence. In its claim to superior knowledge over the empirics, clinical trials internalized the very accusation that the latter bore as a stigma by privileging the role of the experimenter over the medical practitioner in the use of bodies as sham devices or placebos. In our case the covenant, Hunter's reference point for discussing the Shias, was the blindfold, the placebo device; a sham, it nevertheless invoked the idea of the body as a device for arriving at the truth about the Shias through their practices.

In the next section I shall explore the location of the Hooghly Imambara Hospital in the British scheme of improvement that was installed through the processes of appropriation of the Hooghly Imambara endowment over the nineteenth century.

MEDICAL IMPROVEMENT: THE FRONTIERS OF PIETY

In 1806, Haji Mohamed Mohsin willed his property at Syedpore in Jessore for the upkeep of the Imambara. Making endowments after the names of "*waqf-e-awlad*" or "*Waqf-e-khandaan*" in strict conformity with the Sharia was not conventional prior to the Permanent Settlement of 1793.[14] Endowments were rarely willed as such. They became so, no doubt, following the introduction of private property in Bengal that year and the increasing transfer of property in the following years.

Haji Mohamed Mohsin formally bequeathed the Syedpore estate in Jessore (presently in Bangladesh) to promote pious activities associated with the Hooghly Imambara, authorizing his two friends, Rajub Ali Khan and Shakir Ali Khan, to act as Mutawallis. According to the Haji's will, the Mutawallis were to pay the revenue of his estates to the government and divide the rest of the income in nine shares, of which three shares were to be spent on commemorating the auspicous days and festivals organized by the Haji in the Imambara, in the repairs of the Imambara and the cemetery; the two Mutawallis were to appropriate two shares equally for themselves; and four shares were to be spent toward the payment of pensions and stipends of those chosen by the Haji.[15]

After Haji Mohamed Mohsin's death in 1812, the Mutawallis defaulted in revenue payments to the government. In 1819, the government expelled the present Mutawallis, Baker Ali Khan and Wasiq Ali Khan, in accordance with Regulation XIX of 1810, which empowered it to intervene in religious endowments bypassing the court. It was alleged that "the proper objects of the endowment were neglected," and "the income was spent on quarrels between the managers, bribes to the police and *amins*, and gifts to the manager's relatives."[16] The Mutawallis lost their final appeal against the government to the Privy Council in 1835.[17] In 1835, the same year in which Macaulay submitted his *Minute on Education* to the Board of Directors, the governor general of India, "deeming himself to have succeeded to the full authority and power assigned by Haji Mohamed Mohsin to the Mutawalli" became the final arbiter of the fate of the endowment.[18] In 1836, the government founded the Hooghly College from the funds allocated for one of the Mutawallis and invested the part allocated for the payment of stipends and pensions to the construction of a hospital. The college and the hospital came to signify the secular portion of pious activities, and normatively meant for the public. It nominated another Mutawalli, Akbar Ali, for the religious part of the endowment, making him answerable to the government for the collection of rent and expenses incurred in the Imambara.

Significantly enough, while the establishment of the college was deemed controversial in the light of the ongoing controversy between the Orientalists and the Anglicists over the appropriate use of native endowments in education, the legitimacy of the hospital was not questioned; this was so despite the fact that the government had chosen to note that the Haji's will did not explicitly mention any hospital, just as he had not committed any part of the endowment for education explicitly. Effectively, by targeting the will as the site of intervention, the East India Company claimed inheritance to what, following Koslowsky, was a *riasat*, meaning a dominion resembling a kingdom, rather than what the officials claimed—an estate.[19] Endowments such as the Haji's (*waqf Khairi*) were dedicated to the circulation of social goods in the everyday quotidian lives of the faithful through the Imambaras in the form of provisions for madrasahs and *maktabs*, dispensation of medical relief, and payment of salaries and stipends of scholars as well as serving larger symbolic aspirations such as, for instance, supplying weapons to warriors fighting in the path of God and funds for the establishment and maintenance of Imambaras.[20]

But most importantly, the Imambara, through which the services were dispensed, was also the house of the one who founded the endowment, a relationship made explicit by the Haji in his will.[21] Most of the endowment property was territorially too scattered to represent a coherent state—Syedpore in Jessore, which supported the Hooghly Imambara endowment—is today geographically located in Bangladesh. However, the coherence of the activities associated with the Imambara can be made out from the fact that he did not stipulate any funds exclusively for charities in the form of the madrasah, the Unani *dawakhana* (dispensary), or, for that matter, the *bawarchikhana* (kitchen) for the pilgrims and the faithful.[22]

In the final instance, what the British appropriated was the authority to access what was not written in the will. What was not written had been left to the Mutwallis, who had been "tried and approved" by the Haji and found to be "possessing knowledge, religion and probity," to interpret.[23] The afterlife of the will, undergirded by notions of Shia piety as well as personal likes and preferences of the Haji of which the Mutwallis were knowledgeable, was given over to them to interpret. It was also this afterlife of the will over which the Mutwallis Shakir Ali and Wasiq Ali sought to secure their right over by claiming, to the objection of the government, the Haji's deed as one of gift.[24] Entrenched in the world of orality, the will was always in waiting, to be enlivened through remembrance, speech, deliberation rituals, and the politics thereof. It was this world which the British would appropriate in the process of claiming its value as the basis for adjudicating the Mutwallis' failure to pay the revenue.

The British works of improvement were, therefore, installed on a prior understanding of juridical immunity to characterize existing modes of circulation of social surplus as unaccounted for, despotic, and aberrational. No doubt this justification was explained by the government's own initiative to secure the endowment on a profitable footing, which again involved restructuring the political economy of native religious endowments. The account of *jama* (assessed revenue) and *kharch* (expenses) clearly demonstrated proper objects of the endowment had not been addressed. Paradoxically, this claim registered a new way of assessing revenue, whereas under the Mughals the *jama* or assessed revenue, as we know used to be inflated without any intention of mirroring the actual or the *hasil*, which used to be much less.[25] The British would rectify this "discrepancy" between the assessed and the real by imposing a lower revenue rate but insisting on timely payment of the full amount.[26]

The incorporation of the whole endowed estate under the *patni* system followed the government's issuance of Regulation VIII of 1819, which for the first time acknowledged the zamindar's right to lease out in perpetuity. It formalized a system that had been in abeyance in the estates of the Burdwan Raj since 1799. In fact, the *patni* system was embossed in the Burdwan estate soon after the Permanent Settlement, when, having run into revenue arrears and faced with auction the Raja farmed out his property in perpetuity to his employees/tenants, thus repeating on his subjects the same conditions by which he was bound to the government.[27] The investment of hefty advances from the *patnidars* and fines were invested and accumulated, with interest in government securities. In official imagination at least, it registered the government's claim to trusteeship of the Haji's will as legitimate even though the mode of appropriation might not have won approval of British bureaucrats.[28]

Thus, through the procedures of investigation of performance of the Mutwallis in relation to the will, a new code of righteousness was simultaneously produced, which enabled the British government to interfere in the quotidian practices of the Imambara. The Haji had explicitly mandated a part of the ninth share of the endowment for Muharram. Muharram was a collective rite of suffering in which Shia Muslims mourned in procession the martyrdom of the Prophet's grandson Imam Hussain by copiously weeping, beating their breasts, and on occasions wounding themselves with knives or chains.[29] This rite of worship or *ibadat* involved active participation in painful practices in order to cultivate virtuous conduct.

Pain here did not represent the body in passive state, or a renunciation of moral agency but, rather, following Talal Asad, a conscious commitment to acts of worship that had to be promoted through self-discipline as aspects of one's faith.[30] In 1831 the European magistrate set rules for the conduct of Mohurram at Hooghly, which targeted such acts as a potential threat to life itself.[31] These rules explicitly forbade parading the streets with sticks, swords, or arms of any description; against playing native music or drums near European houses; and close surveillance of the procession by police and European soldiers.[32] In other words, the British state in India differentiated Shia faith as one of the singular inspirations of the Haji's will only to authorize itself to classify the associated practices as veritable sites of riot and crime involving disavowal of self-discipline, and similar situations demanding state intervention.

However, this is not to say that the Mohurram had ceased to be present in the calculations except as an event demanding policing; it was decided that Mirza Akbar Alee, the government-appointed Mutawalli, was heretofore

> to wait upon the collector of Zillah Jessore after the ten days of the Mohurram and the completion of the business thereof without delay, to take possession of the mehals and strictly attend to the discharge of the duties of collection and realization and keep the tenants and cultivators contented and thankful by peacable measures, and put the mehals in such regularity and order that the payment of the Government revenue and management of all the concerns may be perfectly affected conformably to the Towleatnamah of the late Hajee Muhammad Mohsin, without any derangement taking place.[33]

This instruction for Akbar Alee initiated the actual appropriation of the endowed estate of Mohamed Mohsin, and the ouster of the Mutwallis Wasiq Ali and Shakir Ali. Muharram clearly continued to matter in marking out the initiation or commencement of appropriative actions as governmental procedures. The plan shows the British state at its acquisitive best, cautiously avoiding the Muharram so as not to provoke sentiments, but moving decisively nonetheless.

Within this discourse of righteousness the hospital found its place as a site of public piety, representing an instrument of circulating the surplus back into the social body. But more importantly, if read in the light of the British policies toward Shia rituals of worship, the hospital came to be seen as the place where the native subjects would be civilized by introducing them to productive pain which claimed relief as its goal. Following this vein of argument, the establishment of the hospital was mandated by the government's perception of practices peculiar to the Shia sect as a source of wasteful, gratuitous pain.

Later in the twentieth century, recounting Badan Chowdhury's achievement in his speech, his son would vouch for the popularity of the Imambara Hospital under Esdaile, drawing as it did people from as far as Delhi.[34] This obscured the already existing connection between the Imambara, Awadh and Persia created by pilgrims, and effectively echoed the general tendency of the government to deny the legitimacy of this connection on suspicion of the Imambara committee's purported proclivities toward wasteful expenditure; this was the case in the late nineteenth century, when a huge group of Shia mourners arrived in the doors of the Hooghly Imambara after the death of Wajid Ali Shah, the exiled Nawab of Awadh, at Metiabruz.[35] It was around this time that the hospital underwent rapid expansion, with the government requisitioning a bigger share of the Haji's endowment for building an operation theatre.[36]

In the next section, I shall study the British pursuit of legitimacy for the Hooghly Imambara Hospital by studying the works of James Esdaile, civil surgeon of Hooghly and principal of the Hooghly Mohsin College.

ESTABLISHING LEGITIMACY: MESMERISM AT THE HOOGHLY IMAMBARA HOSPITAL

Both formal historiography on Victorian subcultures and historiography of medicine in South Asia have explored James Esdaile's experiments with mesmerism in the Hooghly Imambara Hospital.[37] In this section, I shall incorporate the Hooghly Imambara Hospital to understand the Victorian subculture's encounter with its Oriental other in British-ruled Bengal. Thomas Alexander Wise, who was not only the secretary of the local agency and oversaw much of the "appropriation" of the endowment was also deeply committed to the works of improvement and involved in framing future policies for the institutions. Not surprisingly, it was he who made the transfer, semantically and spatially, from the *dawakhana* on the southern part of the Imambara to a place outside it, in a two-storied building. Wise was to lament the failure of the hospital to draw the response from the natives that had expected it would.

However, the appearance of James Esdaile seemed to allay Wise's concerns rather decisively. Records of Esdaile's successes with the native patients have impressed the historians no less than it impressed Lord Dalhousie. His "success" over the native patients over a period of eight months fetched him an invitation to dine with Lord Dalhousie, and the promise from the same of a Mesmeric Hospital in Calcutta. His assistant Badan Chandra Chowdhury was honored with an interview with the governor general.[38] However, back home, Esdaile found himself incapable of putting his countrymen on mesmeric trance; his experiments following his retirement in Edinburgh and London left him disappointed, leading him to reiterate with finality that the natives of India were more susceptible to mesmeric influence.[39] This observation has led me to reconsider the rising flow of native patients in the Hooghly Imambara Hospital in the light of Esdaile's own descriptions of the profile of the patients. They were, in his admission, the "poorest," "most ignorant," "convicted felons of the most degraded order" who produced deep aversion in him. Therefore, it would not be far-fetched to state that Esdaile was carrying out his experiments with mesmeric trance on the prisoners of the Jail Hospital of Hooghly at the Hooghly Imambara Hospital. His own arthritic problems, coupled with the fact that for quite a while he was having to carry out the dual responsibility as the civil surgeon of Hooghly and heading the Hooghly Mohsin College had restricted his mobility beyond the Imambara establishment. This, no doubt, goes a long way in troubling any straightforward acceptance of the government's figures representing the popularity of the hospital under Esdaile.

In fact, Esdaile was fairly candid about the violence involved in his experiments. He allowed skeptical gentlemen to carry pins with them in the theater for testing the strength of mesmeric trance on patients. He was also quite forthcoming about his anxieties centering on his project of creating a public theatre of medical performance. Fighting a lone battle on behalf of mesmerism as a credible anesthesia against surgical pain from the periphery of the empire, James Esdaile left no stones unturned to simulate the conditions of public platforms associated with societies pursuing science in the West. His efforts in his own admission, were aimed at reaching out to the discerning public in England to gather support for his cause.

In one such public demonstration of mesmeric trance on a woman named Gendoo, Dr. Esdaile decided to give in to Dr. Bedford's demand that Muriatic acid be poured on the ulcerous sore covering the right temple of the patient while she was awake. He did so in order to assuage Dr. Bedford of his suspicion that the patient had not been manipulated before the trace. Gendoo's lack of immediate reaction to this infliction made Dr. Esdaile apprehensive. He writes,

> There could be no doubt about it, she was found out! The arch deceiver having set a snare and delusion for me, was now laughing at my beard; and I was not relieved from my thick-coming fancies by Dr. B kindly suggesting, "that she was probably a very insensible person naturally."[40]

Declaring that her head was on fire, she sat up, showing signs of great pain, got out of the bed and walked about distractedly in great agony, screaming that the doctors had put pepper on her and she was on fire. Immediately, Dr. Esdaile had her bathed in cold water, threw her into trance and took this opportunity to pare the tubercles around the sore. Esdaile chose to read these incidents as instantiation of the need to expand his trials with mesmerism. The trials were not merely targeted toward the immediate objective of surgical operation; variation in responses to mesmerism was also reflective of the wide array of circumstances that the mesmerist needed to record, compare, analyze the flow of sympathies from the mesmerist to the patient, and apprehend any future disruptions.

Lokee, a woman whose tumor had been operated upon came back to the hospital on its recurrence. Failing to mesmerize her and having no time to spare, Dr. Esdaile operated on her. Throughout the operation Lokee screamed, crying that she was being murdered and continued to be in great pain hours later. Dr. Esdaile concluded,

> This perverse and inconsistent conduct appears to me to be easily accounted for, from the very fact of her being aware of what was wanted and intended to be done; her anxiety to go to sleep neutralized her good intentions—excitement and mind being destructive of the mesmeric influence for the production of coma.[41]

Under Esdaile, therefore, the Hooghly Imambara Hospital and the jail establishment were brought together, which enabled Esdaile to maintain a clinical distance between him and his native patients, their suffering being reified as a necessary byproduct of the experiments.

Esdaile's desire for public audience in London, mediated by his public demonstrations of vivisection on natives in the Hooghly Imambara Hospital was meant to vindicate his critique of some of the institutions of medical authority, such as the Royal Chirurgical Society of London; the latter, Esdaile complained, had recently allowed Dr. Copeland to declare, without a word of disapprobation, that pain was wise.[42] No doubt, Esdaile was fighting his own battle as a Scot, who was banned by law from practicing beyond the jurisdiction of the Royal College of Surgeons of Edinburgh.[43] Having made his way to the shores of Bengal and survived the tropical heat to bestow the natives with his therapeutic dreams, Esdaile discovered practices familiar to mesmerism present in the ways of life in the form of magic. His eight months in the Hooghly Imambara Hospital allowed him to anticipate the providential meeting between theology and science through his attempts to sieve the scientific basis of mesmerism from the primitive "mummeries" of an archaic belief. This scientific faith was no doubt enabled by the Imambara Hospital in the form of a perfect device for producing consensus between the intentions of the British surgeon and the expected response from the deservedly unfree native. It produced both the threat of mischief, of deception that the practitioner could anticipate from the subaltern, as well as the necessary resolve to overcome it in the next sequence of experiments.

However, this threat of mischief was also symptomatic of a deeper connection between the way medical agency was constituted with its over reliance on surgery to canvass Western medicine in colonial India. No doubt the stress on surgery was historically constituted through the close networks shared by the East India Company and Edinburgh Medical School.[44] But it was these institutional histories echoing the earthly associations between Esdaile and the Hooghly Imambara Hospital and glorifying the conquest of pain in surgery (especially at a time when the Medical College in Calcutta was lamenting not having enough patients in the surgical ward) which gave surgery in British India the necessary historical credibility. Such conquests of surgical pain were realized by anticipating the mischief of the patient—the irritant which contested the planned procedures forced a new route to finally emerge in the records as another novel case of mesmerism.

In 1895, while explaining the unpopularity of the Hooghly Imambara Hospital to the resistance of low-class native parturient women against being used as objects of instruction, Surgeon D. G. Crawford wrote, "The patient may not know whether she is being used for instruction or not, but she probably knows that a (medical) class exists, and *jumps to the conclusion that she is admitted to hospital rather as a subject than as a patient*."[45]

Unpredictable behavior, routinized in official voice, nonetheless betrayed the concern about the native blurring the crucial distinction between the subject and the patient. In his response Crawford unwittingly voiced the ambivalent location of the native woman in relation to the linear historiography of the Western patient, from the tortured soul in medieval ordeals to the desiring subject of modern medicine. Surgeon Crawford's revelation, however, came at the expense of reasserting the salience of remaining intentionally ignorant of the ambivalent location of the native subject in relation to the British works of improvement. Much like the architects of placebo-controlled "blind assessments," he chose to remain resolute in his conviction that such behavior was caused by ignorance.

DAKTARI: STAGING MEDICAL RELIEF

Let us go back to that afternoon at Chinsurah, to the one-storied "masonary" structure, where zamindars, native personnel, and resident invitees of Hooghly had gathered to witness the formal opening of the dispensary in the presence of the civil surgeon of Hooghly, Major E. E. Waters. Speaking about his father, Jogendrolall animated the image of a self-made man who studiously learned the art of mesmerism as an aid to surgery from James Esdaile and went on to attend the sick diligently and with care, without differentiating between the rich and the poor. His disposition toward public piety, Jogendrolall asserted, was not restricted to his medical profession alone; he also internalized the knowledge of medicine in the form of faith through rigorous practices of ascetic abstention in his private life. In support of this claim Jogendrolall said, "A man of regular habits he worked from early morning to dewy eve. . . . A total abstainer from meat and all sorts of intoxicants he was a devoutly religious man and lived a long and simple life, dying at the age of 93."[46]

Soon after, however, Jogendrolall would be reminded of the limits of his expression of filial piety. The Raja of Burdwan opened his speech, saying, "My coming here this morning has been prompted by a duty that I owe to the representative of the family of the late Dr. Budden Chandra Chowdhury in consideration of the esteem and regard in which His Highness the late Maharajdhiraja Maharaja Mahtab Chand Bahadur of Burdwan held the late doctor."[47] In the rest of the speech he explicated the content of this duty by underplaying Jogendrolall's projection of the opening of the dispensary as a mark of his "filial piety." The Raja pointed out that the dispensary was a memorial which Badan Chowdhury had given himself by explicitly registering it in his will. Hence, he asserted, Jogendrolall and his "fellow townsmen of Hooghly," who did not appear to be aware of the qualifications or the merits of the late benefactor, would have to do more in terms of keeping his memory alive. They would have to ensure that the charitable dispensary did not become an "opposition shop" against the interests of the Hooghly Imambara Hospital but rather act as a "helpful and necessary addition to the bigger institution."[48]

Now, the decorum had clearly marked out the hierarchy of speakers. The raja of Burdwan, Jogendrolall's critic, had been "asked" by no less than the major to take the stage. Through his call for distributing medical charity in a "concentrated manner," [49] the raja was giving a formal *nirdeysh*,[50] a direction toward remedying a discordant note represented by the aspirations of Jogendrolall and his supporters in Hooghly. It is true that the Hooghly Imambara endowment had expanded its medical relief beyond the hospitals to other charitable dispensaries in and around Hooghly. Its expansion probably happened in the aftermath of the Burdwan Fever in the 1860s, when there were frequent complaints by British civil surgeons of villagers of the Hooghly district ending up in dispensaries managed by the Burdwan Raja's fund. Thus, Hooghly had become territorially integrated in medical terms through British investment of the endowment funds. However, much of the land in Hooghly had been leased out by the Burdwan Raj in the form of patni tenures. Within these networks of power involving spatial continuities in the form of proprietorial hierarchies on land, and discontinuities in the form of the government's operation of territorially demarcated medical charity, Jogendrolall's claim to the dispensary of Badan Chandra Chowdhury and his aspirations around it appeared to have posed a threat to the sanctity of the Imambara Hospital as the center from which medical poor relief was to be distributed.

Indeed, Jogendrolall's own depiction of his father in an ascetic frame was a claim to the authority of the *daktari* idiom, represented by the body of the self-less medic. Of course, this depiction discounted the fact that the contestations over his right to private practice during his tenure as the assistant surgeon of the Hooghly Imambara Hospital. The signs of a brewing conflict between the Chowdhurys and the Imambara establishment can be traced back to the days when Badan Chowdhury was a salaried employee of the Imamabara. According to George Toynbee, the British magistrate of Hooghly, Keramat Ali, the then Mutwalli, had complained in a petition which was signed not only by Muslims but also by one Hindu, against the native doctor for being "proud and ill-natured," prone to avoid "visiting the sick poor at their homes," and with leaving the hospital soon after the civil surgeon "turned his back." The Mutawalli seemed to have taken severe exception to the fact that much of Badan Chandra Chowdhury's travels in palanquins in relation to his private practice had to be borne by the Imambara. They also stated that they considered his salary to be a "misappropriation of the Imambara funds."[51] The local agents of the government were all too eager to defend Badan Chowdhury and attributed this petition to a general adverse "tide of feeling" among the Mahomedan community. Toynbee, too, appears to have lent his weight in support of the doctor. He had to depend on Badan Chowdhury's testimony for his description of the Imambara prior to its reconstruction in 1864. Badan Chowdhury, too, did not hesitate to lend his weight against the Mutwalli in the official register. He called the expansion of the structure, which Akbar Ali, the Mutwalli, had initiated, as "waste of money."[52] In the light of these preexisting discordant notes, Jogendrolall's aspirations no doubt forced the Raja of Burdwan to caution him against invoking his "filial piety" to ends that went against the "concentrated" medical relief. *Daktari* had thus emerged as a political platform on which contests for power would be staged.

CONCLUSION

The memorialization of Badan Chandra Chowdhury was part of a broad economy of remembrance that sought to stabilize his afterlife by keeping at a remove or disciplining the notes that were not consonant with the existing status quo between private wealth and public charity. Evidently, in such contestations of the status quo in the context of the early twentieth-century phase of the nationalist movement, the image of the ascetic doctor was a powerful symbol. This study was undertaken to understand how this image achieved the representational power that it did. To this endeavor I have located the memorialization of Badan Chowdhury as the vantage point to understand how medical relief was constituted as a necessary work of improvement through the appropriation of the Hooghly Imambara endowment.

It is noteworthy that British commitment to the cause of improvement through the Haji's endowment and its claim to the trusteeship also produced a decisive shift in the existing pedagogic culture of the Muslims. The Anglicist Orientalist debate of the 1830s, which had concluded with the plan to "engraft"[53] the natives with Western arts and sciences through Persian, Arabic, and Sanskrit, was finally negotiated, in view of administrative exigencies, in favor of introducing Bengali as the vernacular medium of translation. Even as John Stuart Mill advocated continuation with the existing seminaries of education against Anglicist plans of transplanting English, he could not but state that "mischief" within such institutions as sufficient cause for their reform. The Hooghly Mohsin College, incidentally, was the institution chosen to highlight Bengali, a dialect that the Muslims purportedly abhorred to study.[54] The introduction of a Bengali class at the Medical College at Calcutta further underscored the government's plans on vernacularization of education.

Hence, the conversion of the *dawakhana* within the Imambara to a hospital outside it was part of a much broader project of appropriation and social mediation of the production of agrarian surplus enabled by the government's control over the will of the Haji. Following the above study, the pre-history of *daktari* or the constitutive moment of juridical immunity to intervene on and elicit imagination of a therapeutically united vernacular/national body was conditioned by the appropriation of religious endowments on the one hand and the development of a classificatory vision of labor in colonial imagination on the other. In 1852, George Campbell would identify the "rising class of Hindoos," "especially of the mercantile and the writer classes" as "hard working" vis-à-vis the Mahommedan respectable families, who had served the offices of the rulers for generations and would have been extremely suitable for British administration but for their tendency to live in "reminiscences of past greatness."[55]

The history of the emergence of native medical labor for the civilian population in British India had complex origins in so far as it was introduced as part of a broader installation aiming at social mediation. In its aspirations to cleanse the mischief of the Haji's endowment and establish an alternate idea of productive pain, the British government introduced the hospital as a sanitary space, enjoying juridical immunity to intervene corporally. It is, I argue, important to think of how this corporal immunity reconfigured the role of mediating the instability associated with quotidian practices of reciprocal gift giving within the Shia community—a role until now represented by the world of the Imambara.[56] The conflict between Badan Chandra Chowdhury and the Imambara establishment over private practice vis-à-vis public duty was symptomatic of the authority that medical agency emerged to claim for itself over the latter half of the nineteenth century within the Imambara establishment while representing the broader scheme of British-governed medical relief. Ironically, it was the inauguration of Badan Chowdhury's dispensary, a self-memorial the latter had willed before death, which was chosen as an occasion to launch medical relief as a platform for claiming political legitimacy on behalf of the collective body.

NOTES

1. I use the word "fragmentary history" to underline the sinews of difference represented by minority cultures, which tend to be appropriated by the unifying claims of liberal, Brahminical, Hindu, nationalist mainstream history writing. See Gyanendra Pandey, "In Defense of Fragment: Writing about Hindu-Muslim Riots in India Today," *Representations* 37 (1992): 27–55.
2. I am indebted to Dr. Swapan Ganguly for providing me with the excerpt from Dr. Badan Chowdhury's *Dispensary Records* titled "The Opening Ceremony of Dr. Budden Chandra Chowdhury's Outdoor Charitable Dispensary." (1913).
3. See Waltraud Ernst, "Colonial Psychiatry, Magic and Religion: The Case of Mesmerism in British India," *Psychiatry* 15, no. 1 (2004): 57–71. While Ernst rightly questions the clear-cut boundaries between science and magic through her case study of the career of mesmerism and the reasons for its ostracization by the British government, she ends up reifying the binary by claiming a scientific status for mesmerism that was purportedly denied to it by the "scientific establishment" because of its "heterodoxy." My chapter questions this binary and seeks to locate it within a broader history of vivisection and placebo.
4. "The Opening Ceremony," 6.
5. Situated on the bank of Hooghly River, Bhatpara is known for its rich traditions in the field of Sanskrit learning. The name "Bhatpara" originates from the ancient name Bhatta-palli where "Bhatta" denotes the name of Brahmin Sanskrit Pundits and "palli" denotes a locality or village. en.wikipedia.org/wiki/Bhatpara (last modified 25 June 2011).
6. "The Opening Ceremony," 1.
7. W. W. Hunter, *The Indian Musalmans* (New Delhi: Indological Book House, 1969, 1871), 113.
8. W. W. Hunter, *The Indian Musalmans*, 112.
9. Fazlur Rahman, *Islam* (London: Weidenfield and Nicholson, 1966), 172–73.
10. Ted J. Kaptchuk, "Intentional Ignorance: A History of Blind Assessment and Placebo Controls in Medicine." *Bulletin of the History of Medicine* 72, no. 3 (1998): 389–443.
11. Edward Gibbon, *The History of the Decline and Fall of Roman Empire*, vol. 2 (1840): 402–3.
12. W. W. Hunter, *The Indian Musalmans*, 113.
13. Ted J. Kaptchuk, "Intentional Ignorance: A History of Blind Assessment and Placebo Controls in Medicine." *Bulletin of the History of Medicine* 72, no. 3 (1998): 389–443.
14. G. C. Kozlowski, *Muslim Endowments and Society in British India* (Cambridge: Cambridge University Press, 1985), 40.
15. Francis Bradley-Birt, *Twelve Men of Bengal in the Nineteenth Century* (Lahiri, 1910), 47–50.
16. Bradley-Birt, *Twelve Men*, 52
17. Bradley-Birt, *Twelve Men*, 53
18. Bradley-Birt, *Twelve Men*, 54

19. Kozlowski, *Muslim Endowments and Society*, 47.
20. Kozlowski, *Muslim Endowments and Society*, 1.
21. Bradley-Birt, *Twelve Men*, 47.
22. Letter no. 11 dated 2 January 1836 from the Govt. of Bengal to the Sudder Board of Revenue, *Collection of Papers Relating to the Hooghly Imambara, 1815–1910*, 173–76.
23. Bradley-Birt, *Twelve Men*, 48
24. Sudipta Kaviraj, "Writing, Speaking, Being: Language and the Historical Formation of Ideas in India," in *The Imaginary Institution of India: Politics and Ideas* (New York: Columbia University Press, 2010), 132. As Sudipta Kaviraj has pointed out, it is important to remember that the British introduced writing as a dominant mode of ratification of agreements in a society which was predominantly mnemonic. Mnemonic reproduction, which allowed for slippages, inadvertence, and interpretation with or without deliberate intent allowed flexibility within a formally rigid structure, affording those who directed society considerable space for informal amendments.
25. Under the Mughals *jama* was more a statement of hopeful expectation than of actual tax receipts. "The Mughals and their ilk were extortionate, but they did face some constraints. In their time India still had a great deal of unoccupied land. Peasants often move when pressed too hard. Cultivators. Zamindars and village headmen became adept at concealment and resistance. All of these limited the ability of pre-British states to get every *rupee* they asked for." See G. C. Kozlowski, *Muslim Endowments and Society in British India*, 86.
26. Ibid.
27. W. W. Hunter, *A Statistical Account of Bengal*, vol. 4 (London: Trubner and Co., 1876), 79.
28. The peculiarity of the case of Hooghly Imambara came up for discussion in relation to the question of repealing Regulation XIX of 1810. House of Commons Papers, vol. 40, *On Hindu Idolatory and Mohametanism* (1849). The mode of appropriation of the Hooghly Imambara endowment also came up for severe criticism by the Legal Remembrancer. See Letter no. 2034 dated 15 October 1863 from C. P. Hobhouse, Superintendent and Legal Remembrancer to the Government of Bengal, 1863, 363–66, *Collection of Papers Relating to the Hooghly Imambara, 1815–1910* (Calcutta: Secretariat Book Depot, 1914), 9.
29. Two different types of processions took place during Muharram. The first imitated Imam Husain's march toward Karbala. These had a distinctly military aura featuring armed men, drummers, and trumpeters with some marchers carrying banners of martial insignia. This procession served to remind onlookers of Husain's courage and prowess. The second type of procession recreated the burial of Husain and his followers. During this phase of the ritual, replicas of their tombs, also called *taziyah*, were carried through the streets and taken to a field outside the city. The participants took the *taziyah* to a field called "Karbala" and buried the ones specially built for the occasion. Both the processions and the *majalis* provoked intense emotions. See G. C. Kozlowski, *Muslim Endowments and Society in British India*, 28–30.
30. For an elaborate discussion on the relationship between bodily pain and Islamic practices, see Talal Asad, *Formations of the Secular: Christianity, Islam and Modernity* (Stanford: Stanford University Press, 2003), 108.
31. George Toynbee, *A Sketch of the Administration of the Hooghly District from 1795 to 1845* (Calcutta: Bengal Secretariat Press, 1888), 131.
32. Toynbee, *A Sketch of the Administration*, 131.
33. *Sanud* dated 15 November 1816, from Board of Revenue to Syed Akbar Ali Khan appointing him as ameen to take charge of the Syedpore Esate and the Institution at Hooghly, *Collection of Papers*, 27.
34. "The Opening Ceremony," 8.
35. Letter no. 189, 19 August 1898, from the members of the committee for the management of the Hooghly Imambara to the Revenue Dept. Govt. of Bengal, *Collection of Papers* (1914), 605–10.
36. Letter no. 379T, 7 June 1899, from the Govt. of Bengal to the Board of Revenue, *Collection of Papers* (1914), 630.

37. Alison Winter, *Mesmerized: Powers of Mind in Victorian Britain* (Chicago: University of Chicago Press, 1998). From the point of view of South Asian medical historiography, see Waltraud Ernst, "Colonial Psychiatry, Magic and Religion: The Case of Mesmerism in British India." *Psychiatry* 15, no. 1 (2004): 57–71.

38. "The Opening Ceremony," 8.

39. "Esdaile," *The Indian Medical Gazette* 36 (1906): 464.

40. Esdaile, *Mesmerism*, 52.

41. Esdaile, *Mesmerism*, 89.

42. Esdaile, *Mesmerism*, 7.

43. Medical practice was governed by provincial guilds in Great Britain until 1858. See Lisa Rosner, *Medical Education in the Age of Improvement: Edinburgh Students and Apprentices, 1760–1826* (Edinburgh: Edinburgh University Press, 1991).

44. Lisa Rosner, *Medical Education in the Age of Improvement: Edinburgh Students and Apprentices, 1760–1826* (Edinburgh: Edinburgh University Press, 1991).

45. D. G. Crawford, *Hooghly Medical Gazetteer* (Calcutta: Bengal Secretariat Press, 1902), 311

46. "The Opening Ceremony," 5–6.

47. "The Opening Ceremony," 9.

48. "The Opening Ceremony," 11.

49. "The Opening Ceremony," 10.

50. *Bengali and English Dictionary for the Use of Schools* (1856).

51. Toynbee, *A Sketch of the Administration*, 141.

52. Toynbee, *A Sketch of the Administration*, 140.

53. The word "engrafting" had its theological roots in Calvin's normative prescriptions of being united with Christ in the sixteenth century. Represented by the iconography of the vine and the vine grower, Calvin had invoked the Holy Spirit as the actual agent of "engrafting" of the faithful with the spirit of Christ by enabling the subject to articulate his faith in the form of knowledge. The Holy Spirit was associated with the *work* of "engrafting" the subject by preventing him from being led astray by magic. The act of "engrafting," Calvin had stated, was regenerative or restorative in so far as the subject pledged to be led by the example of Christ's life, thus committing the self to the force of punishment. This is instructive because, following Agamben, the Church Fathers introduced the Greek word *oikonomia* in the theological discourse as the divine economy between the second and sixth centuries CE in order to endorse the Trinity as a "practical" problematic. The Church's claim that God was threefold in nature caused perturbations among the faithful (later called monarchists) anxious to avoid polytheistic influences. It was now that theologians came up with the word *oikonomia* as a distinct realm from that occupied by the God in substance. Unlike the latter, he administered and governed his home, life, and the world that is the *oikonomia* as triple. Hence, engrafting, in so far as it represented the subjectification of the person to the norms of the Calvinist monastic order in the sixteenth century, was itself a practical activity iconized by the Holy Spirit, distinguishing the orientation of the act as predominantly praxis of faith achieved through noetic (vis-à-vis mystical) experience. See Sung-Sup Kim, "Engrafting: The Image of Union in Calvin's Commentary on John's Gospel," *Journal of Reformed Theology* 4 (2010):112–28. Also see Giorgio Agamben, *What Is an Apparatus? and Other Essays* (Stanford: Stanford University Press, 2009), 1–24.

54. The Muslims of Hooghly found a Bengali language to be a "dialect of no dignity and of little use." For details, see K. Zachariah, *History of Hooghly College 1836–1936* (Bengal Government Press, 1936), 32.

55. George Campbell, *Modern India: A Sketch of the System of Civil Government to Which Is Prefixed Some Account of Natives and Native Institutions* (London: John Murray, 1852), 291.

56. Here I read the medical immunity as reconfiguring what Roberto Esposito identifies as the inherently unstable nature of gift giving by claiming a disciplinary control over the very bodies which produced the agrarian surplus, the basis of British revenue in India. See Roberto Esposito, "The Immunizing Paradigm." *Diacritics* 36, no. 2 (2006), 23–48.

Chapter Five

Colonial Medicine and Elite Nationalist Responses in India

Conformity and Contradictions[1]

Shamshad Khan

In my earlier work on systems of medicine and mainstream nationalist discourse in colonial India, I outlined three major streams in the nationalist discourse—conformity, defiance, and quest for an alternative.[2] Based essentially on the United Provinces (UP) Assembly proceedings, private papers, official documents, and archival materials, my study revealed that while the elements of conformity to biomedicine and the Western system of knowledge remained more pronounced and emphatic, those of defiance were conversely weak and at times even apologetic. The quest for alternatives—largely represented by Mahatma Gandhi—on the other hand, although powerful and able to build trenchant civilizational and institutional critique of modern science and medicine, could never find adequate space in the national agenda for social change. I also argued that although the "cultural authority" and hegemony of biomedicine over indigenous science and knowledge was initiated by the colonial state, it was extended by the mainstream national leaderships and national governments with far more extensive and profound implications and less resistance.

This chapter, drawn on the same set of historical sources, examines the tensions, ambiguities, and ambivalence within the nationalist discourse on medicine and health and within the voice of conformity to biomedicine. It also demonstrates, in particular, that while as a way of contesting colonial authority and as a mark of Indian nationalism, the national elites of India tried to revitalize the Indian systems of medicine, especially Ayurveda and Unani, these efforts were equally entangled with class, communal, and religious politics, often polarizing the debates. Ironically, polarizations along lines of group and sectional interests—some of them based on old, primordial relations—were very much part of the same discourse on modernity, science, and progress which dominated the debate on the revitalization of Indian medicine. This chapter holds that these tensions and contradictions in the modernization debate on medicine and health in India, especially as reflected through the mainstream national politics in the late 1930s and 1940s, militate against the hegemonic claims of universality (that is, speaking for the nation) by elite Indian nationalists.

ON RATIONALE, METHODS, AND SOURCES

This chapter is in the mold of a critical policy and discourse analysis. As a case study, it focuses mainly on the proceedings of the United Provinces Legislative Assembly from the late 1930s and 1940s and, where relevant, makes use of private papers, official documents, and archival materials. It holds that examining assembly debates from the late 1930s and 1940s is critical to understanding elite nationalist responses to colonial authority, including colonial medicine and public health. This is important for several reasons. As a result of the constitutional reform brought by the Government of India Act 1935, the Indian National Congress (INC), the main organizing nationalist body, had won an absolute majority in provincial legislatures in 1937, and formed the first mass-elected representative governments in seven out of eleven provinces, including UP.[3] Being in power at the provincial level, the Indian nationalist leaders were virtually the policy makers and could significantly shape future policies and programs, including those related to public health and medicine. Recognizing their role and the fact that by the 1930s the chances of India getting political freedom had become quite imminent, the INC had also instituted a National Planning Committee (1938) to prepare blueprints on various issues for what it felt would be a planned change after 1947.[4] Although findings from the proceedings of the UP Legislative assembly cannot be claimed to represent the complexity of nationalist discourse on medicine and health in India, given the historical significance of UP in shaping India's national and democratic politics, the legitimacy and significance of the voices and trends emerging from here cannot be overemphasized.[5]

It is important that while in the last few decades there has been a surge of interest in the medical history of India under colonial rule, most of these studies have remained primarily confined to the nineteenth century and focus on colonial medical interventions and their sociopolitical implications.[6] Although the hegemonic and universalistic claims of Indian national elites have long been exposed by critical scholars, especially those engaged in subaltern studies,[7] few works in the realm of history of medicine in India have engaged in such an analysis.[8] Indeed, except for Jeffery's *The Politics of Health in India*, there has been no substantive effort to examine the mainstream nationalist agenda on medicine and health in India.[9] Similarly, hardly any literature exists on issues governing government policies, as reflected through assembly proceedings and debates. It is in this context that this research becomes extremely important.

SOCIAL CLASS, ALLOPATHY, AND REVITALIZATION OF "INDIAN MEDICINE"

As anti-imperialist agitations against the British rule in India grew into a mass movement, and as the calls for *swadeshi* and *swaraj* became more widespread—giving birth to simultaneous demands for boycott of foreign goods, national education, and village and national reconstruction, etc.—the pressures on the mainstream nationalist leaders to include indigenous systems of medicine, mainly Ayurveda and Unani, in the nationalist program also increased.[10] Indigenous medicines were widely popular and culturally integrated in Indian society. In the absence of allopathy, which remained closely associated with the colonial state and largely confined to "colonial enclaves" as well as metropolitan elites, these systems were also often the only options available to Indian people, especially at the grassroots level.[11] Indeed, given the proximities of Western medicine with the colonial state and its dominance, any lack of recognition and inclusion of indigenous medicines in the nationalist program would have jeopardized the very legitimacy of the national movement.

Thus, by the 1920s, the Indian National Congress passed its first resolution in favor of the indigenous systems of medicines,[12] and when the Congress-led ministries were formed in the 1930s, this led to government-sponsored efforts toward their revitalization at the provincial level. In UP, for example, the first mass-elected nationalist government passed "The United Provinces Indian Medicine Bill, 1938."[13] The main aim of the Bill was "to provide for the development of the Indian systems of medicine and to regulate their practices in the United Provinces."[14] A more detailed analysis of the provisions of the bill and the nature of the debate in the assembly that followed reveals that the effort was mainly to professionalize and "modernize" the Indian systems of medicine with allopathy taken as the idealized model. It was proposed, for example, to establish teaching and research institutions and laboratories and to develop the art of surgery based on the allopathic system. It was also proposed to reconstitute the Board of Indian

Medicine—originally founded in the 1920s, but largely ineffective—as a *statutory* and *representative* body to coordinate the system of medical education and training, the system of examination, and the granting of degrees, aid, and funds. Besides, there was a proposal to root out "quackery"—considered a "menace"—from the practices of the Indian systems of medicine. This, it was argued, could be achieved through a regulation of the system of appointment of vaids and hakims in the government services and in private practice. However, despite these efforts toward revitalization, the Indian national elites were never fully convinced of the value of the indigenous systems of medicine. In fact, most of them believed that the indigenous systems could never be a match to allopathy—which was viewed as "modern," "scientific," evidence-based, and effective—and, therefore, should not be given a priority or equal treatment in the nationalist agenda for social change. For example, Atmaram Govind Kher, the parliamentary secretary to the minister of Local Self-Government and Health, Vijaya Laxmi Pandit, believed that allopathy was more advanced and superior as it had new ways of diagnosis, such as radiology, the new art of surgery, and modern surgical instruments as well as bacteriology, all of which were absent from the indigenous systems of medicine.[15] He also added that allopathy should not be discriminated against on the ground of being foreign because, to him, knowledge did not belong to any particular country; it was and should be treated as "universal science," irrespective of its place of origin.[16] Kunwar Sir Maharaj Singh, a member in the assembly, although in favor of the revitalization of Indian systems of medicine, openly declared his own preference for the allopathic system: "Personally I am in favor of the modern or allopathic system of medicine."[17] Similarly, Raja Jagannath Baksh Singh, another member, stated: "However much effort may be made for its progress, the Indian systems of medicine cannot be a match to the Western system."[18] Begum Abdul Wajid even suggested that money being spent on Ayurvedic and Unani colleges should be diverted to allopathic medical colleges.[19]

It is important to note that these were not simply individual opinions expressed in the assembly, but instead were very much a part of the dominant discourse and both reflected as well as shaped government policy. A major chunk of government grants, for example, went to allopathy. Raghunath Vinayak Dhulekar, a member of the Legislative Assembly, reported that out of two and a half crores[20] spent annually on health in UP, only five to six thousand rupees were granted to the colleges of indigenous medicine, and fifty thousand each to Banaras Hindu University and Aligarh Muslim University; the rest was spent on allopathy.[21] There might be some exaggeration in his estimate, but it certainly gives us a fair idea of the major difference in monetary support to indigenous and Western systems of medicine. Similarly, in terms of employment, Ayurvedic and Unani graduates were rarely appointed to the posts of medical officer in the Provincial Medical Service and never to the higher posts, such as that of inspector general of Civil Hospital. They were also mainly employed in rural areas, while allopathic doctors remained urban based.[22] When concerns were raised against the "discriminatory" policy of the government vis-à-vis appointments, Vijaya Laxmi Pandit, minister of Local Self-government and Health, stated that vaids and hakims lacked "background" and sufficient "fundamental education."[23]

It appears that the ground for this kind of unequal or discriminatory policy vis-à-vis different systems of medicine was partly created by the National Planning Committee, an important organ of the Indian National Congress. For example, a key member of its Sub-committee on National Health, Dr. J. C. Ray, notes:

> There have been attempts in this country during recent years to give a semblance of science to indigenous systems of medicine by providing laboratories and dissection of human bodies, etc. But the correct course should be to accept the large body of scientific knowledge in Western medicine as the nucleus round which only the scientifically tested knowledge derived from the indigenous systems of medicine should grow. . . . The scheme of training which we should adopt, therefore, should be unprejudiced by considerations of sentiment, and should be based solely on scientifically tested knowledge.[24]

Jawaharlal Nehru, who headed the National Planning Committee in the 1930s and later became India's first and long-serving prime minister with huge influence on its institutional building, had similar views:

> The science of medicine would not be divided up into compartments but would be built upon solid foundations of past and present experience tested by modern scientific methods. . . . The proper approach, therefore, should be that any system of medicine to be followed or encouraged must be modern and up-to-date and should take advantage of all the accumulated knowledge we possess.[25]

Clearly, to Nehru and to most of his colleagues in the National Planning Committee, indigenous systems of medicine were less than a "science" and far from modern Western science, which they must pursue in order to receive any government support or encouragement. Indeed, at a deeper level, it sounded not much different from the approach adopted by the colonial state, which insisted on scientific evidence of safety and efficacy from the indigenous systems of medicine and "privately . . . believed that to place these systems on a scientific basis would be to destroy them utterly."[26]

Much of the faith in Western science and medicine or lack of confidence in the indigenous systems of knowledge, as shown by Indian nationalist elites, could be understood in terms of their internalization of the dominant colonial discourse. As Arnold points out, by the late nineteenth century, Western medical ideas—deeply mediated by colonial discourses—had begun to "infiltrate and inform public debate and political language to a quite remarkable degree."[27] But this had also to do with their deep-rooted class interests. India's mainstream national leaderships, as also reflected in the UP Legislative Assembly, mainly composed of the rich and urban middle classes, most of whom were Western educated. Many of these members or their families had been patrons and active consumers of Western medicine and they obviously did not want to lose their privileges.[28] Yet, revitalizations of Indian medicine received support from them, because besides providing legitimacy to the national movement—and placating demands from vaids and hakims—these were also deemed necessary to meet the urgency of unmet needs for medical care in rural areas. The 1946 *Report of the Health Survey and Development Committee* (also called the Bhore Committee report), for example, had pointed out high morbidity and mortality levels in rural areas and a severe lack of institutional care, especially in UP. According to the report, the average rural population served by one medical institution in UP was 105,626, and the average number of villages to be served by a medical institution was 224.[29] Vijaya Laxmi Pandit also reported in the assembly that while indigenous systems of medicine were sufficiently popular, culturally integrated, and, above all, cheap, the allopathic system was too expensive and beyond the reach of the rural population.[30] Thus, moved by urgency and compelled by its own financial constraints, the ministry had no option but to fall back on the indigenous systems to fill the gap. I argue that responding to the "pressure from below" in an ad hoc manner, where only a half-hearted support was provided to the indigenous systems, perpetuated the colonial legacy of a discriminatory and fractured health system: that is, one for the army and British civilians, which was later extended to the rich and urban middle classes, and another for the poor and marginalized, especially in the rural areas which remained largely neglected. The Indian national elites could have played a more balanced role in truly integrating the indigenous and Western systems of medicine, perhaps along similar lines as experienced in China. Regrettably, the practice of maintaining the hegemonic position of allopathy at the cost of indigenous systems of medicine has continued as a part of the dominant ruling class ideology.[31]

SYSTEMS OF MEDICINE AND RELIGIOUS AND COMMUNAL POLITICS

It is paradoxical that even in the midst of the debate over modernization of Indian medicine and the utmost concern for modern scientific knowledge, Indian nationalist discourse was riddled with religious, communal concerns. Thus, Ayurveda and Unani were polarized on communal lines, frequently associated with Hindus and Muslims. And, questions were raised regarding the representation of Muslims in allopathic colleges as well as dispensaries. Measures for vaccinations and sanitations were also opposed, or guided along religious, communal lines. For example, when the proposal was made that six members (out of twenty-five) of the new Board of Indian Medicine would be elected from among the vaids and hakims based on their proportional representation (in the Board's Register) and joint electorate, several Muslim members in the house rose in opposition asking for equal representation and separate electorate for the hakims. Their fear was that proportional representation and a joint electorate would hamper Unani as a system of knowledge and science and be unfair to hakims, who were numerically less in number compared to vaids. Zahiruddin Farooqui wondered

> whether the government is going to allot seats on the basis that both systems are treated as science or on the basis of number of vaids and hakims, or the number of Hindus and Muslims in the province. Now I put to the government that even if all the Muslims in this province became Hakims, they will [*sic*] at the most command only 15 percent. . . . If the Board is composed on the basis of population, it would not be fair.[32]

Similarly, Muhammad Ishaque Khan suggested that in terms of representation the government should maintain equality between the two systems of medicine so that the Board "may command universal confidence." He also cautioned that proportional representation might lead to corruption through bogus registration (for acquiring seats on the Board) and that joint electorate would not be proper as it would be difficult for vaids and hakims to know the representative qualifications of each other.[33] Although not without merit, these questions and concerns were reflective of the tensions within the revitalization efforts and the call for Indian medicine.

Another communally charged exchange occurred over the fate of Jarrahs. These were traditional Muslim folk surgeons found predominantly in Western UP, who were considered "unqualified" and because of the regulation to control "quackery"—a part of the Indian Medicine Bill—were going to be adversely affected. Against this regulation, Zahiruddin Farooqui moved an amendment whereby he wanted Jarrahs to be excluded. However, this amendment was defeated. The pattern of the votes cast shows that out of eighty-three votes against the amendment, only three were Muslim votes, while out of twenty-three votes in favor of the amendment suggested by Farooqui, all were Muslim votes.[34]

There were similar polarizations over the United Provinces Mela Bill—this bill sought to regulate religious fairs and gatherings for the sake of sanitation, hygiene, and public safety—over the issue of appointments of vaids and hakims in newly established dispensaries, and over the issue of community-based admission of students to allopathic medical colleges in

UP. For instance, A. B. A. Haleem (a member in the assembly) protested against the low number of Muslim students and teachers at the Agra medical college, and wanted to know what steps the government proposed to secure a fair allocation for Muslims in the matter of admission and representation on the staff of the college.[35] Ishaque Khan, another member, pointed out that there was a "universal dissatisfaction" among the Muslims against the procedures for selection adopted by the Agra medical college.[36] He also inquired about the number and names of the male nurses employed by the Civil Sadar Hospital, Basti, during the last three years, and sought to know why no Muslim was taken in 1936–1937, and what the reasons were for the paucity of Muslim Compounders and male nurses.[37] In 1939, when twelve Indian dispensaries were opened in rural areas and vacancies were announced for 146 vaids and forty-six hakims, Tahir Hussain enquired about the reason behind a considerable difference in the number of vacancies for vaids and hakims. He showed displeasure when told by Atma Ram Govind Kher, the secretary to the minister of Local Self-government and Health, that the difference was according to their ratio in the register maintained by the Board of Indian Medicine.[38] Similarly, S. M. Rizwan Allah wanted to know the community-wise list of the number of students who had been admitted to and graduated from King George Medical College, Lucknow, since its inception.[39] Thus, although on the one hand there was a general enthusiasm to use modern, Western scientific standards to Indian systems of medicine, on the other hand, this enthusiasm was quite often influenced by religious, communal questions and concerns. They were very much part of the same discourse.

It should be noted that, historically, both as knowledge systems and in terms of their practice and access, Unani and Ayurveda have neither been static nor aloof, and never strictly confined to Hindus and Muslims. Their dynamism and syncretism, in general, and fruitful interactions with each other in particular, are well documented.[40] However, from the assembly debates, it appears that the nature of interaction between the two systems changed and remained tense over the decades of the 1930s and 1940s. Leslie (1976, 1992), Jeffery (1988), and Quaiser (2001) too have uncovered elements of internal conflict and tensions within and between Unani and Ayurveda.[41] This was clearly linked with power struggles, the issue of institutional control and dominance, and with the larger sociopolitical environment in the country around the demand for Pakistan and India's partition. This goes further to demonstrate that science and medicine are contested terrains constituted by and constitutive of politics, ideology, and culture; the universalistic claims of Indian national elites—that is, speaking for the nation or Indian medicine —were far from reality.

This chapter, thus, offers a grounded critique of the elite national politics and discourse on medicine and health in colonial India, especially as reflected through assembly debates and policies during the late 1930s and

1940s. It holds that examining assembly proceedings from the late 1930s and 1940s is critical to understanding elite nationalist responses to colonial authority, including colonial medicine and public health. This is especially so in view of the importance of these two decades for India's modern institutions and given the shortage of literature on systems of medicine and nationalist discourse.

Drawing on assembly proceedings, private papers, and official documents, this chapter reveals that the mainstream Indian nationalists were never fully convinced of the value of the indigenous systems of medicine. In fact, most of them believed that the indigenous systems of medicine could never be a match to allopathy and, therefore, should not be given a priority or equal treatment in the nationalist agenda for social change. This faith in allopathy or lack of confidence in the indigenous systems of medicine resulted in discourses, policies, and practices that overwhelmingly favored Western medicine with only a modicum of support for the indigenous systems, thereby perpetuating a colonial legacy of subordination and subservience of indigenous systems of knowledge. This chapter has also highlighted that while much of the fascination of Indian national elites for modern Western science and medicine could be understood in terms of their internalization of the dominant colonial discourse as well as the dictates of building a modern nation-state, it had also to do with their deep-rooted class interests. As at least partially reflected in the United Provinces Legislative Assembly, most of the mainstream Indian nationalists belonged to the rich and urban middle classes and were active consumers of Western medicine, a privilege which they did not want to lose. However, they also recognized and provided some support to the indigenous systems, as they were deemed necessary in light of the urgency of unmet needs for medical care among the rural poor and the marginalized as well as sociocultural and political imperatives of leading a national movement.

Finally, this chapter has demonstrated that despite its zeal for conformity to modern Western science and rationality, the Indian nationalist discourse on medicine and health was not completely free from religious, communal politics. Indeed, class, communal, and religious polarizations were very much part of the modernization debate on medicine and health in India and had votaries who spoke simultaneously—often through ambivalence and forked tongue—for universal science, modernity, nationalism, and their own sectional interests, some of these interests and stakes flowing from old primordial relations.

This critique of nationalist discourse on medicine and health in no way justifies or rehabilitates colonialism and its aftermath. It rather emphasizes the need to adopt a critical stance to both colonialism and nationalism, for it is only through our reflexive critique that solutions to much of our postcolonial misery may be found.

This chapter is based on my deep commitment to critical pluralism, which, while appreciative of the coexistence of varied medical traditions, equally insists on exploring and examining networks of power, domination, and hegemony which actively shape and constitute those relationships. Such a framework, I believe, has the potential to achieve a truly existing medical pluralism and an integrated system of medicine.

NOTES

1. Excerpts of this chapter have previously been published in my article "Systems of Medicine and Nationalist Discourse in India: Towards 'New Horizons' in Medical Anthropology and History," *Social Science and Medicine* 62 (2006): 2786–97.

2. See Shamshad Khan, 2006; Also see Shamshad Khan, *Medicine, Health and Nationalist Discourse in Colonial India, 1937–1947*, Unpublished thesis submitted to Jawaharlal Nehru University, New Delhi, 1994.

3. The INC had won absolute majorities in five provinces—namely, UP, Bihar, Central Provinces, Madras, and Orissa—and the largest single party status in four provinces. For details, see D. Gupta, *Indian National Movement* (Delhi: Vikas Publications, 1970). Also, see Sumit Sarkar, *Modern India 1885–1947* (Madras: Macmillan India Limited, 1983).

4. This National Planning Committee had twenty-nine sub-committees formed into eight groups and with special terms of reference to deal with all aspects of the national life.

5. UP has historically been the most populous province in India, with huge influence on political processes, and has had the largest number of India's prime ministers originating from here.

6. See for example David Arnold, "Medical Priorities and Practice in Nineteenth-Century British India," *South Asia Research* 5, no. 2 (1985): 167–83; David Arnold, *Colonizing the Body: State Medicine and Epidemic Disease in Nineteenth-Century India* (Berkeley, University of California Press, 1993); David Arnold, *Science, Technology and Medicine in Colonial India* (Cambridge: Cambridge University Press, 2000); Radhika Ramasubban, "Imperial Health in British India, 1857–1900," pp. 38–60 in *Disease, Medicine, and Empire*: *Perspectives on Western Medicine and the Experience of European Expansion*, edited by Roy MacLeod and Milton Lewis (New York: Routledge, 1988); Rajnarayan Chandavarkar, "Plague Panic and Epidemic Politics in India, 1896–1914," pp. 203–40 in *Epidemics and Ideas*: *Essays on the Historical Perception of Pestilence*, edited by Terence Ranger and Paul Slack (New York: Cambridge University Press, 1992); Poonam Bala, *Imperialism and Medicine in Bengal*: *A Socio-historical Perspective* (New Delhi: Sage Publications, 1991); Mark Harrison, *Public Health in British India*: *Anglo-Indian Preventive Medicine*, *1859–1914* (New York: Cambridge University Press, 1994); Biswamoy Pati and Mark Harrison, eds., *Health, Medicine and Empire*: *Perspectives on Colonial India* (New Delhi: Orient Longman, 2001); Deepak Kumar, "Unequal Contenders, Uneven Ground: Medical Encounters in British India, 1820–1920," pp. 172–190 in *Western Medicine as Contested Knowledge*, edited by Andrew Cunningham and Bridie Andrews (New York: Manchester University Press, 1997); Anil Kumar, *Medicine and the Raj*: *British Medical Policy in India, 1835–1911* (New Delhi: AltaMira Press, 1998).

7. See, for example, edited volumes of *Subaltern Studies*: *Writings on South Asian History and Society* (Delhi: Oxford University Press). Ranajit Guha was the editor of the first five volumes from 1982 to1989. Also see Ranajit Guha, *Elementary Aspects of Peasant Insurgency in Colonial India* (New Delhi: Oxford University Press, 1983); Ranajit Guha, *Dominance without Hegemony: History and Power in Colonial India* (Cambridge: Harvard University Press, 1997).

8. Arnold's *Colonizing the Body* (1993) has a chapter on "health and hegemony," broadly delineating "resistance, accommodation and appropriation of Western medicine" by Indian middle-class leaderships and elites; however, it is focused mainly on the nineteenth century.

Also see Gyan Prakash, "Body and Governmentality," in his book, *Another Reason: Science and the Imagination of Modern India* (Princeton, NJ: Princeton University Press, 1999). Prakash seems to exaggerate the strategies of "reinscription" (and their subvertive value) used by Indian national elites in dealing with colonial governmentality, including colonial medicine and therapeutics. He also ignores class. Also see K. N. Panikkar, "Indigenous Medicine and Cultural Hegemony: A Study of the Revitalization Movement in Keralam," *Studies in History* 8, no. 2 (1992): 283–308; Poonam Bala, "'Defying' Medical Autonomy: Indigenous Elites and Medicine in Colonial India," pp. 29–44 in *Biomedicine as a Contested Site: Some Revelations in Imperial Contexts*, ed. Poonam Bala (Lanham, MD: Lexington Books, 2009); B. D. Metcalf, "Nationalist Muslims in British India: The Case of Hakim Ajmal Khan," *Modern Asian Studies* 19, no. 1 (1985): 1–28; Charles Leslie, "The Ambiguities of Medical Revivalism in Modern India," pp. 356–67 in *Asian Medical Systems: A Comparative Study*, edited by Charles Leslie (Berkeley: University of California Press, 1976); Debabar Banerji, "The Place of Indigenous and Western Systems of Medicine in the Health Services of India," *Social Science & Medicine* 15A (1981): 109–14.

9. Roger Jeffery, *The Politics of Health in India* (Berkeley: University of California Press, 1988).

10. At individual and group levels, vaids and hakims, some of them prominent nationalist leaders such as Hakim Ajmal Khan, were already working toward the revitalization of Indian systems of medicine. For more details along this line see Metcalf, 1985; K. N. Panikkar, 1992; Also see Paul Brass, "The Politics of Ayurvedic Education: A Case Study of Revivalism and Modernization in India," pp. 342–71 in *Education and Politics in India*, edited by S. H. Rudolf and L. I. Rudolf (New Delhi: Oxford University Press, 1972).

11. Arnold, 1993; Radhika Ramasubban, *Public Health and Medical Research in India: Their Origins under the Impact of British Colonial Policy* (Stockholm: SAREC, 1982); McKim Marriott, "Western Medicine in a Village of Northern India," pp. 239–68 in *Health, Culture and Community: Case Studies of Public Reactions to Health Problems*, edited by B. D. Paul (New York: Sage Foundation, 1955).

12. Jean Langford, *Fluent Bodies: Ayurvedic Remedies for Postcolonial Imbalance* (Durham: Duke University Press, 2002).

13. *The Proceedings of the Legislative Assembly* (United Provinces, India, 31 March 1939), 94–109.

14. *The Proceedings of the Legislative Assembly*, 94.

15. *The Proceedings of the Legislative Assembly* 31 (1947): 96.

16. *The Proceedings of the Legislative Assembly* 31 (1947): 96.

17. *The Proceedings of the Legislative Assembly* 16 (1939): 49.

18. *The Proceedings of the Legislative Assembly* 31 (1947): 489–90.

19. *The Proceedings of the Legislative Assembly*, 486–87.

20. A "crore" in Indian currency is equivalent to ten million.

21. *The Proceedings of the Legislative Assembly* 31 (1947): 481–82. Both Banaras Hindu University and Aligarh Muslim University had separate departments of Ayurveda and Unani medicine.

22. *The Proceedings of the Legislative Assembly*, 487–88.

23. *The Proceedings of the Legislative Assembly*, 487–88.

24. National Planning Committee, *National Health* (Report of the Subcommittee) (Bombay: Vora and Company Publishers, 1948), 58–59.

25. *Selected Works of Jawaharlal Nehru* 14, pt. 2 (New Delhi: Orient Longman, April–July, 1950): 288–89.

26. Roger Jeffery, "Allopathic Medicine in India: A Case of Deprofessionalization?" *Social Science and Medicine* 11 (1977): 570.

27. Arnold, *Colonizing the Body*, 280.

28. Arnold (1993) and Bala (2009) also deal with patronage and support provided to Western medicine by Indian elites (especially Parsis, Hindus, Muslims) as part of strategies of accommodation and buying influence, prestige as well as political recognition from the colonial regime.

29. Government of India, *Report of the Health Survey and Development Committee* 1 (Delhi: Manager of Publications, 1946), 35–38.
30. *The Proceedings of the Legislative Assembly* 16 (1939): 49.
31. R. Frankenberg, "Allopathic Medicine, Profession, and Capitalist Ideology in India. *Social Science & Medicine* 15A (1981): 115–25; Also see Debabar Banerji, 1981, "The Political Economy of the Introduction of Western Medicine in India and Pre-existing Health Services," *International Journal of Health Services* 39, no. 4 (2009): 803-9.
32. *The Proceedings of the Legislative Assembly* 18 (1939): 439.
33. *The Proceedings of the Legislative Assembly*, 442.
34. *The Proceedings of the Legislative Assembly*, 484–88.
35. *The Proceedings of the Legislative Assembly* 26 (1947): 26; Also see 3–4.
36. *The Proceedings of the Legislative Assembly* 26 (1947): 26; Also see 3–4.
37. *The Proceedings of the Legislative Assembly* 4 (1938): 366.
38. *The Proceedings of the Legislative Assembly* 12 (1939): 82–83.
39. *The Proceedings of the Legislative Assembly* 13 (1939) 97–98.
40. See M. Ali, "Ayurvedic Drugs in Unani Materia Medica," *Ancient Science of Life* (1990): 191–200; A.L. Basham, "The Practice of Medicine in Ancient and Medieval India," in *Asian Medical Systems* (1976): 18–43; Charles Leslie, "Interpretations of Illness: Syncretism in Modern Ayurveda," pp. 177–208 in *Paths to Asian Medical Knowledge*, edited by Charles Leslie and A. Young (Berkeley: University of California Press, 1992); Panikkar, 1992.
41. Leslie (1976, 1992); Jeffery (1988); Nishat Quaiser, "Politics, Culture and Colonialism: Unani's Debate with Doctory," pp. 317–55 in *Health, Medicine and Empire*: *Perspectives on Colonial India*, edited by B. Pati and M. Harrison (New Delhi: Orient Longman, 2001).

Chapter Six

Colonial Compassion and Political Calculation

The Countess of Dufferin and Her Fund

Seán Lang

Few British medical initiatives in India were as riddled with paradox and apparent contradiction as the celebrated fund to "supply Female Medical Aid to the Women of India" launched by the Vicereine, the Countess of Dufferin, in 1885. In theory, the Countess of Dufferin's Fund, as it was usually known, was a national association of women's hospitals, training courses, and female medical schemes spread throughout the Indian Empire, all under the general direction of the Fund's Central Committee in Calcutta; Lady Dufferin herself usually referred to "The National Association" and stressed its uniquely India-wide reach. In reality, the association was a very loose federation and its authority over its regional branches depended entirely on their willingness to accept it. Bombay was notorious for disregarding instructions from the Central Committee, though other branches did so on occasion, and there was little Fund officers could do about it except to write ever more mordant comments in annual reports.[1]

The Fund attracted extravagant praise both in Britain and in India, but this was seldom matched by the scale of donations, so that it was constantly short of money; the low pay and relatively poor employment conditions in Dufferin hospitals became notorious.[2] The language of female emancipation was central to its rhetoric, yet the Fund formed the basis of a Women's Medical Service for India specifically designed to be subordinate to the existing one for men.[3] Fund literature boasted of its exclusively female hospitals, yet it was administered at the top almost entirely by men and its hospitals were open to inspection by male medical officers.[4] It can even be argued that the

Fund's role was more political than medical. It conducted itself as an organ of state, proudly boasting that it owed its foundation "to the direct initiative of the Queen-Empress" and that it hoped its work would strengthen the political bond between Britain and India.[5] Viceroys and provincial governors presided over the Fund's public ceremonies; its administrative officers and council members were drawn from within the viceroy's staff; its Central Committee met at Government House and wrote its correspondence on government notepaper. Successive vicereines found themselves expected to assume the presidency of the Fund whether they wanted to or not. From the moment it was founded, the Countess of Dufferin's Fund was part of the political and administrative fabric of the British Raj.

Unlike most British colonial medical initiatives, the Countess of Dufferin's Fund was aimed at the perceived medical needs of the indigenous population rather than those of Europeans. Moreover, it was posited on the idea that its work would strengthen the ties not only between India's women and their European "sisters," but also to their distant "mother," the queen-empress. The real measure of its success, therefore, would lie less in its medical work than in the responses it prompted among the Indian population, and especially among Indian women. It is these responses that this chapter will seek to gauge.

THE MAHARANI'S MESSAGE

The Fund's administrators were well aware that Western intervention in indigenous practice in female medicine might provoke an adverse reaction. The risk had been well illustrated by the celebrated episode which first highlighted the issue for many in Britain and India, the message sent to Queen Victoria in 1881 by the Maharani of Punna. The Maharani gave her message, concealed in a locket, to the Church of England medical missionary Elizabeth Beilby to give to the queen.[6] It appealed for women doctors to be sent from England to work with Indian women living in seclusion. The story fitted perfectly the popular Western image of India as an exotic land of secluded damsels in distress and it was immediately seized upon by medical missionary groups looking for support.[7] The episode has also been taken by historians as prima facie evidence of official sanction for the whole "medical women for India" movement from the British political establishment.[8] The full story, however, is both more complex and more revealing.

At first, the audience appeared to go well. The queen noted in her journal that "Miss Beilby gave a melancholy account of these poor ladies" and that she had expressed her "deep interest and hope that something might be done in this matter."[9] In the guarded language of the court, this was a strong sign of royal approval and it prompted immediate rejoicing in the missionary press.[10] The palace was surprised to learn, therefore, that shortly after the audience Beilby left the Church of England mission; she angrily denounced it for amateur medical standards, leaving its London central committee with no choice but to accept her resignation.[11] More alarming was the news of the very angry reaction to the audience that was reported from the Maharajah of Punna. Like any Indian ruler, the Maharajah was conscious of the importance of maintaining respectful relations with his queen-empress; he had met the Prince of Wales during his tour in 1875 to 1876 and had been presented with the gold badge and ring, distributed as a mark of favor to minor rulers, along with a rifle, a claymore, and, intriguingly, a corridor fire engine.[12] The giving of gifts in Indian princely society was calculated with great care, and the Maharajah would have been well aware that his wife had put the queen-empress in her debt by the gift of the locket. He was reportedly angry that it should have contained a message for the queen, about which he knew nothing, and he was particularly agitated to learn that the Maharani had allowed Beilby to pray within the precincts of his Zenana, something which he did not permit, and even that his wife had apparently expressed an interest in knowing more about Christianity.[13]

Palace officials were disturbed when they learned of the Maharajah's reaction, especially since it soon appeared that the Maharani's reported interest in Christianity had been wishful thinking on Beilby's part.[14] If a pro-British figure like the Maharajah could be angered in this way, the possibility of over-eager missionaries giving widespread offense by interfering in the women's quarters of Indian households and claiming to do so with royal approval was truly alarming. Under the circumstances, it was thought fortunate that sending a framed photograph of the queen to Puna, intended as a reciprocal present in acknowledgement of the locket, had been delayed; it was thought wisest to let the matter quietly drop.[15]

THE FOUNDING OF THE COUNTESS OF DUFFERIN'S FUND

In the aftermath of the Beilby audience the crown made it very clear that it would support the rapidly growing movement to provide female medical help for India only if it was kept rigidly separate from missionaries. The queen noted to her private secretary, "The Queen *does* support the Medical Women for India as else they die for want of any help—*but* not to connect this *with Religion at all*."[16]

In October 1884, the queen recommended to the Countess of Dufferin, who was visiting Balmoral with her husband before leaving for India, that she might look into the issue of Indian women's health. She did not mention the Beilby audience and neither woman mentioned the issue in their diaries, which might suggest that it was not discussed in any detail or depth, but there is no reason to doubt that the conversation took place; it took place, moreover, within a highly politically charged context.[17] Lord Dufferin had been appointed to the viceroyalty specifically to repair what was generally seen in Britain as the damage done by his predecessor, the liberal reformist, Lord Ripon. Ripon had sponsored the ill-fated Ilbert Bill, a proposal to allow some categories of European defendants to be tried before Indian magistrates, which, to the dismay of Indian nationalists, had been withdrawn in the face of general outrage among the European population. Inter-community relations in India were, therefore, in a delicate state by 1884 and the queen, who had been appalled by the Ilbert Bill, was well aware of it.[18] She welcomed the appointment of Dufferin, whom she knew well, to reverse Ripon's Liberal agenda. As consort and vicereine, it was Lady Dufferin's duty to support her husband in this task, and it is in this political context that her high-profile, state-approved medical charity needs to be viewed.

Lady Dufferin's correspondence with the queen shows that the idea of a national organization only took shape in her mind when she had had the chance to familiarize herself with existing arrangements in India. She found that, while important schemes were up and running in the major cities, they hardly touched India's extensive country districts. In June 1885, Lady Dufferin wrote to the queen about an idea for some sort of "Association" for promoting the Female Medical Question, with a central committee at Calcutta and local committees in the provinces. [19] Her reference to "the Female Medical Question" shows that she was thinking in essentially political terms: "Question," as in "Irish Question" or "Eastern Question," was the standard Victorian term for a thorny social or political issue. Her idea was not to set up an individual female hospital, as had been done in Madras and Bombay, but to set up a network of committees based on the administrative capital and operating mainly through the wives of provincial governors. It was a scheme that neatly reflected her viceregal role and status.

The launch of the Fund was fixed for August 1885 and a draft prospectus was drawn up to explain its scope and purpose: (1) to provide medical tuition for Indian women as doctors and hospital assistants; (2) to provide female-run hospitals, dispensaries, and wards; and (3) to supply trained nurses and *dais* (traditional birth attendants). In the printed version the word "dais" was replaced by "midwives" to remove any impression that the Fund sanctioned traditional Indian birthing practice.[20] The main target of the Fund was to cater to high-caste "purdanashin" women, that is, women living in strict seclusion; in this way, the Fund reflected the way in which Victorians commonly imagined conditions in the East as a whole. After a round of fund-raising garden parties and fancy fairs, the Fund was officially launched with an impressive ceremony presided over by the viceroy: the queen-empress's patronage was confirmed and Lady Dufferin announced that the queen had made a personal donation of £100; the news had been held back from the London papers to increase the impact of its announcement in India.[21] The queen's money was to be used to provide gold medals for the best students at India's five female medical schools, linking her visibly with the movement to improve women's health and, it was hoped, bonding her ever more closely to her Indian peoples. As one local Indian newspaper put it:

> This act of the sovereign is but another instance of the great and unceasing regard she has for all her Indian subjects, and her deep solicitude for their well-being. . . . it will go far to strengthen, if possible, more than ever before the attachment of the people of this country to the Throne of England. . . . Native grandees and others will now be anxious more than before to support that cause and thus show themselves worthy *lieges* of their sovereign.[22]

In political terms, the Fund provided a channel for direct contact between individual Indians and their still recently created queen-empress. The queen's photograph adorned the walls of Dufferin hospitals and wards, various of which were named after her or after other members of the royal family. Visiting or—better—opening women's wards or hospitals became a regular feature of the ceremonial work of viceroys, provincial governors, and visiting royals. The Fund's 1887 Golden Jubilee booklet made it clear that it was carrying out the direct and heartfelt wishes of the queen-empress toward her Indian "children."[23] A special Jubilee subscription to the Fund brought in five *lakhs* (500,000) of rupees, the list of donors being inscribed in a special book that was sent off to the queen. Unfortunately, a majority of the Jubilee subscription came in large, royal eye-catching donations rather than in the less glamorous but more useful form of regular subscriptions to underwrite the day-to-day costs of the Fund's wards and hospitals.[24] Nevertheless, the Fund continued to place heavy emphasis on these high-profile ceremonial events. The annual presentation to the viceroy of the Fund's annual reports, published by the royal booksellers, Hatchard's of Piccadilly, became an important date in the Indian political and social calendar. The reports' usually upbeat details and photographs of hospitals or groups of Indian medical students and pupil nurses reassured readers that Britain's mission to "rescue" India's women was well in hand. The Countess of Dufferin's Fund had become, in effect, the conscience of the Raj.

INDIAN RESPONSES TO THE COUNTESS OF DUFFERIN'S FUND

The political purpose of the Fund would stand or fall on its reception by the Indian population. The most obvious way to gauge this was by attendance at Dufferin hospitals. This, however, was a relatively crude and imperfect method: hospitals tried to keep a record of the precise caste group to which patients notionally belonged, but they found it difficult to make clear distinctions.[25] Although high attendance figures were naturally welcomed by the Fund, on their own they give no clue as to the significance of women choosing a Dufferin hospital over a missionary or government one. More direct evidence is provided by ceremonial addresses to Lady Dufferin, many of them made on the occasion of the Dufferins' departure from India in 1888, and by comment on the Fund in the Indian press. Ceremonial addresses present difficulties of evaluation and interpretation. They were often presented on behalf of "the Women" of a particular place, and were usually written in a florid, adulatory style. They were usually produced by women in the upper echelons of society, but who drafted them and by what process they came to be compiled, is much harder to be sure of. They were written to please: some were preserved by Lady Dufferin in her papers. However, this does not in itself mean that their sentiments were insincere: they did come, after all, from exactly the sort of high-caste women the Fund was hoping to serve.

Newspaper comments, on the other hand, were, usually, written by men and much of it was tied to a more general nationalist agenda. The British certainly took close note of hostile press comment: the vernacular press was regularly perused and summarized for the viceroy; Lord Dufferin took special interest in it. Where ceremonial addresses tended to focus on the medical and educational benefits women got from the Fund, newspaper comment was almost entirely about the Fund's structure and the implications of its work for Indian aspirations for greater autonomy. Indian comment on the Fund concentrated on five main areas which is the focus of the discussion in the following pages: (1) missionaries and religion; (2) the purpose of the scheme; (3) Lady Dufferin herself; (4) the Fund's procedures for appointing medical staff; and (5) the relationship between the Fund and the state.

RELIGIOUS REACTION TO THE FUND

An early reaction in the press was to suspect the Fund of being a front for further missionary activity. Lady Dufferin was herself personally supportive of missionary medicine and was at first happy to employ missionary doctors in Fund hospitals.[26] The Bengal paper, *Bharat Mihir*, a constant critic of the

Fund, hearing that the Dufferin Hospital in Allahabad would be run by an American missionary, commented, "no public measure in this country, it seems, can remain without the pale of European intrigue."[27] Ironically, on this issue the nationalist press was in accord with the queen, who made her opposition to any contact between the Fund and missionaries very clear, as soon as she learned that Lady Dufferin had started to allow them to be employed.[28] The policy was immediately reversed, which, in turn, attracted outspoken criticism from medical missionaries, who accused Lady Dufferin of "gagging" the Fund's Christian employees and dismissing them if they ever spoke of their faith.[29] In an occasional terse correspondence with missionary critics, the honorary secretary pointed out that the Fund was a secular organization, whose officers were appointed "on exactly the same understanding with regard to religious questions as every other Indian official."[30] Opposition from missionaries, some of it very outspoken, was wounding to Lady Dufferin on a personal level, but it had the effect of helping to calm nationalist fears on the issue.

The argument with the missionaries did not affect the Fund's long-term appeal to Indian Christians who continued to dominate its nurse- and medical-training courses. By 1916, for example, they accounted for eighteen out of the thirty-four Fund-supported female students studying at Madras Medical College.[31] However, the willingness of Indian Christians to make use of Dufferin hospitals placed the Fund in a dilemma, since nothing was more likely to deter Hindu or Muslim women than the presence of Indian Christian staff or patients.[32] Indian Christians were usually regarded as renegades by Hindus and Muslims, and their manner did not always endear themselves even to missionaries. One Punjab medical missionary wrote that:

> [Indian Christian patients] "bounce" into the hospital, push in front of the others, and are often indignant when they are told to wait their turn. Often too they are deceitful, and get a lot out of one on false pretences.[33]

The Fund was caught in an identity trap: it sought to be secular, but it operated in seclusion according to what it understood to be Hindu and Muslim practice. Inevitably, this made it appear anti-Christian; at the same time, its links to the state meant that even secluded wards were open to inspection by male government medical officers. Trying to please a range of constituencies, it ended by wholly pleasing none.

The other religious issue confronting the Fund in its early days was whether female medicine was itself sanctioned by Hinduism. Some argued that, as it was not specifically advocated, it should not be encouraged. Shailajanund Ojhah, high priest of the temple at Vaidyanath, published a pamphlet which reasoned that, although female medicine was not actually commended in sacred texts, it was not prohibited either, and that they offered evidence of women having engaged in a healing role. His conclusion was that Lady Dufferin's work had "divine inspiration" and that Rajahs and other leaders of society should support it, so that "no obstacle should bristle up on her way."[34] His verdict was welcomed in the Bengal press for laying out the issue clearly; it was also welcome news to Lady Dufferin, who sent a copy of the pamphlet to the queen, commenting that it "will I daresay be useful," adding, however, "I think some of it will amuse Your Majesty very much."[35] The British had a generally low opinion of Hinduism and especially of its priests: the very problem of seclusion that the Fund was created to mitigate was usually seen as a symptom of an excessively priest-dominated culture. Even the high priest's "useful" pamphlet seemed, to British eyes, to reflect the problem as much as it helped to solve it. Having urged Indians to support the Fund, he went on to urge the Fund itself to recognize the worth of indigenous medicine, pointing out that "if the whole science had been a trashy one, the native physicians of Calcutta would not have been so much in request."[36] He argued that any medical colleges the Fund might establish or support should have chairs in indigenous medicine. Not surprisingly, this proposal found favor in the nationalist press; it was less likely to command respect among Europeans. Some European doctors had respect for indigenous knowledge of local pharmacology, but few thought much of Indian surgery or gynecology; the whole medical women for India movement was predicated on the idea that Indian doctors would not do much good even if they were allowed into the zenana. It seems likely that it was this detail that Lady Dufferin thought would so amuse the queen.

THE PURPOSE OF THE FUND

On the whole, Indian critics did not attack the need for some sort of state-backed initiative to address female health. The nationalist, *Ananda Bazar Patrika*, thought the scheme would greatly benefit the country; *Praja Bandhu*, no friend to the Dufferin administration, thought that Lady Dufferin had "earned the gratitude of the whole nation."[37] However, there was some scepticism about whether the scheme would work. *Samvád Prabhákar* thought that few high-class women would attend Dufferin hospitals and that the Fund would be better employed developing female education.[38] However, none of these newspapers questioned the basic idea that Indian women stood in need of medical aid and that traditional forms of care, especially in childbirth, could not be allowed to continue unmodified. The Bengali *Dacca Prakash* had argued for a government midwifery training scheme back in 1881 and the Calcutta paper *Sanjivani* published in 1886 a vivid account of traditional birthing, calling on the "Christian Government of India" to stop sitting idly by and do something to find "the causes of these evils and to try to prevent their recurrence."[39] *Bhárat Mihir* found it "difficult to describe in adequate terms the beneficial character of the difficult and costly work which Lady Dufferin has undertaken."[40] Such positive comments from a press which was often vehemently critical of her husband was a sign of the challenge posed by Western female medicine to nationalists who wanted to protect indigenous traditions from Western interference: at least in the short term, they simply did not have an answer to those Europeans who pointed to the medical implications for women of living in seclusion.

As the Fund's work got under way, nationalist comment shifted to its impact on other aspects of traditional culture. *Dainik-o-Samáchar Chandriká* and *Navayuga* both protested against criticism by European medical women of the custom of child-marriage; *Sanjivani* entered into a virtual war of attrition with the management of the Lady Dufferin Hospital in Calcutta, denouncing the Fund for accepting women of low repute as pupil nurses and midwives: "the statements of a Committee," it commented acidly, "who can take dancing girls in this country for respectable women should be accepted with care."[41] However, such criticism actually played into the government's hands. It portrayed traditionalists as bigoted, backward-looking, committed to retaining oppressive and unacceptable practices, and thereby served to confirm in British minds the wisdom of keeping Dufferin institutions in Western hands for the immediately foreseeable future.

THE COUNTESS OF DUFFERIN

Much of the adulation the Fund generated was centred on the person of Lady Dufferin herself. Part of this came from her character, which achieved a combination of the elevated and the approachable. Her Indian Journal was published under the lofty title *Our Viceregal Life in India* and showed her in its frontispiece wearing her crown and viceregal sash; the text, on the other hand, revealed her sense of humor and conviviality.[42] She earned the good opinion of the nationalist press early on when it was announced that she was setting about learning Hindi; apart from a few grumbles that she ought to learn Bengali as well, this was generally taken as an encouraging sign of goodwill.[43] Her image also benefited from her easy access to the queen; the constant reminders that the queen had herself originally suggested the issue of female medicine to Lady Dufferin merely underscored the close relationship the two women enjoyed. The position of viceroy was more than a merely representative one; in his official capacity he acted in the place of the monarch, taking precedence even over the Prince of Wales.[44] With a female monarch, however, this concept was easier to conceive through the figure of the vicereine and from the language of ceremonial addresses, many of which referred to Lady Dufferin as "Mother," it seems that for many Indians, Lady Dufferin in effect *was* the queen. Even the most sceptical responses to the announcement of the Fund thanked Lady Dufferin for her initiative and recognized the purity of her intentions. However, some press comment highlighted the inherent fragility of a charity based so heavily on one person. The Bengal newspaper *Sádhárani* pointed out that Lady Dufferin would only be in India for a maximum of five years and asked what would happen to her scheme after she had gone.[45] There could be no guarantee that her successors would take it up with the same devotion and some newspapers feared that her hospitals would eventually be taken over by the government and become Europeanized, like the Eden Hospital in Calcutta, which had been financed by contributions from the community but was largely staffed and attended by Europeans.[46]

Indian responses to Lady Dufferin and her fund were put into perspective in 1888 when Lord Dufferin unexpectedly announced his resignation. This immediately prompted the nationalist press to denounce his government for having achieved nothing of note except to invade Burma and put taxes up. In these circumstances, praise for Lady Dufferin became a way of hitting at Lord Dufferin. The *Dacca Gazette* commented that "though Lord Dufferin has done no good to the people of India, still his name will be associated with that of his benevolent wife and the fund she has opened."[47] *Sanjivani*, whose support for the Fund was almost as consistent as its criticism of the government, even suggested that it might be a good idea to set up a statue of Lady Dufferin rather than one of her husband.[48] The reaction of the Indian press confirmed the idea at the heart of the Dufferin Fund, that its significance lay at least as much in its political role as it did in the quality of its medical work.

No doubt, more welcome to Lady Dufferin herself were the addresses presented to her at the numerous farewell ceremonies she attended after the announcement of her imminent departure. Many of these were given as speeches and then issued in printed form, but some were more elaborate, written on poster-sized paper, decorated with coats of arms or, in the case of one address, from women in Lahore, printed in gold on blue silk. Their language and tone were adulatory. The Lahore address assured Lady Dufferin that she had "a place in our hearts among the noblest and greatest heroines of the past"; one from Punjab found that "words fail to express our admiration of the promptings of your tender and merciful heart."[49] Another from Gujarat stressed the analogy with motherhood:

> Oh mother! The honor and veneration which we attempt to show to Thee fall far short of the true affection cherished by Thee for the people of India. But a good mother never forsakes her children, however undutiful they may be. It is therefore our firm belief that India's well-being will always remain uppermost in Thy mind.[50]

Ceremonial addresses should not be dismissed as mere flummery: they can reflect genuine feelings and they usually show what the writers think will be an acceptable message to the recipient. The Lahore address referred specifically to the retreat of "prejudices against medical treatment on the European lines," which had formerly been "rampant among us," before the "progress of scientific education," which suggests that the women were aware that the Dufferin Fund was intended as part of a more general transformation in women's lives within Indian society.[51] In reply, Lady Dufferin stressed that it was "peculiarly the duty of every woman, no matter how secluded her life may be, to study these questions, to use all her influence to forward these objects."[52] As a political wife herself, she was keenly aware that "far from being invariably downtrodden and helpless, the native woman often rules not only a family but a State, and can from the seclusion of the zenana make her influence very sensibly felt."[53] She was herself an example of how much could be done from a formally constrained position, as some of the addresses recognized. The Lahore women were sure that "Your Excellency's noble and benevolent exertions . . . must have told heavily upon Your Excellency's constitution and health"; the Punjab women spoke of "the sacrifice of every hour of your leisure since you first came amongst us."[54] Lady Dufferin is thus presented as a sort of role model: a hard-working woman who could exert herself in a good cause even to exhaustion within the confines of her role as vicereine, wife, and mother. This ideal of radical change through moderate means was characteristic of the Dufferin Fund's whole approach; it was reassuring to the more cautious among the Indian community and it marked the contrast between the Fund's outlook and the more forceful and energetic style of missionaries and feminist medical women.

FUND PROCEDURES AND APPOINTMENTS

The increasing awareness among Indian commentators by the 1880s of the need for a healthy race and the growing importance in nationalist discourse of the image of *Bharat Mata* (Mother India), served to give an extra political edge to the issue of maternity and female medicine.[55] The overpowering need to save life meant that nationalists were happy to drop the traditional *dai* in favor of the trained midwife or woman doctor, but they expected as many of these midwives and doctors as possible to be Indian. An important theme in criticism of the Fund, therefore, was that it continued to appoint Europeans to fill its vacancies. *Dacca Prakash* was adamant that the money paid into the Fund by Indians should be used to support Indian doctors, and that only so many English doctors should be brought out as would be necessary to establish female medical education.[56] *Bheri* feared that, once Lady Dufferin had gone, English women doctors "will monopolize all high appointments under this scheme."[57] *Sanjivani* objected to the Fund's classification system, which placed women doctors trained in Calcutta below those with European or American qualifications. "Many people entertain the suspicion," it said, "that The National Association is most concerned to provide employment in this country for European female doctors, and that suspicion is likely to be strengthened by the classification of female doctors made by that Association."[58] One Indian doctor wrote to the Fund's Central Committee, "the exclusion of qualified Indian medical women from the highest grade of appointments at the disposal of the National Association is not only unjust, but it would act most injuriously in the way of their professional advancement as private practitioners."[59] In a sense, such criticism was a sign that the Fund had succeeded in its aim of influencing Indian opinion: critics did not want less Western medicine to be available; they just wanted more Indians to be administering it.

Less reassuring for the Fund was criticism of the quality, conduct, and morals of its medical staff. The Fund was accused of bringing out women who knew nothing of midwifery. *Dainik-o-Samáchar Chandriká* described European women doctors as "half-educated ladies . . . a good-for-nothing lot, [who] are not likely to do any good to this country," who charged exorbitant fees and "apparently think that the virtue of protecting women is a monopoly of the British nation."[60] Criticism of the Fund's Indian medical students and pupil midwives was even harsher. *Sanjivani* claimed that women of bad repute were being admitted into midwifery training courses at the Campbell Medical School and that, in any case, medical training under the Fund took far longer than it needed to because of the need to have everything translated.[61] The colorful tone and language of these criticisms should not detract from their valid points: Western-trained doctors and midwives could charge high fees, and the Fund certainly shared in a general European assumption that philanthropy was essentially a Western characteristic.[62]

THE DUFFERIN FUND AND THE STATE

"It is true that Government interest and aid were not wanting," wrote the Allahabad *Pioneer* in 1886 of women's medicine in India, "but the reformation aimed at would have suffered rather than gained by help which in any way savoured of despotic benevolence."[63] This neatly encapsulated the Fund's central problem: how to gain the advantages that came from being linked to the state without appearing to employ state coercion. The Fund's close relationship with the state led some Indians to think it was in fact an official body and the press carried reports of police officers and local officials extracting compulsory donations by force.[64] Even without this overt compulsion, as one paper put it, raising money by public subscription at the behest of the Vicereine of India "amounts practically to the imposition of an indirect tax upon the Indian people."[65] Some newspapers objected to the 1887 Jubilee Fund, which was to be divided between the Imperial Institute in London and the Dufferin Fund. *Samaya* urged that "*Not* one *cowrie*" should be given to either cause, but that money raised by Indians should be expended in India on Indians.[66]

The officials who enforced subscriptions to the Dufferin Fund could be forgiven for their mistake, for by the 1890s, the precise relationship between Fund and state was less clear than ever. Its hospitals were treated as state institutions, their work was inspected and included in annual reports by government medical officers and some were even in the habit of calling in male government civil surgeons to carry out operations, which completely defeated the purpose of an all-female medical service.[67] The precise boundary between the Fund and the state, however, was of more immediate concern to Europeans; for Indians, the ambiguity presented them with an opportunity, by working or studying under the auspices of the Fund, to play a vital role in the operation of an agency whose central importance to the Raj the British themselves stressed repeatedly.

In conclusion, the Countess of Dufferin's Fund was an intensely political organization. Although activated by genuine compassion for the plight of Indian women, especially the suffering many of them went through in childbirth, its ultimate aim was as much to change Indian attitudes toward Western medicine and toward British rule as it was to save life. To an extent it succeeded: it undoubtedly helped to raise the public status of women's health and to establish even in nationalist quarters the primacy of Western midwifery and obstetrics. It also created a strong and widespread attachment to the person of Lady Dufferin herself, an attachment which lasted long after she had left India. The vicereines who followed her found that the presidency of the Fund had become in effect an *ex officio* position. However, nationalist opinion was able to absorb the implications of the Fund and even turn its importance into an argument for increasing Indian and decreasing European participation in its work. Ultimately, the Fund created both a bond between India and Britain and the justification for dissolving it.

ABBREVIATIONS

BLAAS: *British Library African and Asian Studies Collections*
BMJ: *British Medical Journal*
Jnl. NIA: *Journal of the National Indian Association*
MSA: *Maharashtra State Archives* (Mumbai)
PRONI: *Public Records Office of Northern Ireland*
RA: *Royal Archives*

ACKNOWLEDGMENTS

I acknowledge with thanks the gracious permission of Her Majesty Queen Elizabeth II to reproduce material from the Royal Archives and I thank Interserve for granting permission to use material from its Church of England missionary archives.

NOTES

1. *PRONI*: D.1071.J/G/7A/4/C; *MSA*: Bombay *General Department Proceedings* 1903, vol. 29, no. 291; *Eighth Annual Report of the National Association for Supplying Female Medical Aid to the Women of India, 1892* (Calcutta, 1893), 18; *PRONI*: D.1071.J/G/7C/1, Press Clippings File: *Times of India*, 15 March 1897.

2. Maneesha Lal, "The Politics of Gender and Medicine in Colonial India: The Countess of Dufferin's Fund, 1885–1888," *Bulletin of the History of Medicine* 68, no. 1 (Spring 1994): 29–66.

3. See Margaret Balfour and Ruth Young, *The Work of Medical Women in India* (London/New York: Oxford University Press, 1929).

4. *BLAAS*: P/V 492 *National Association for Supplying Female Medical Aid to the Women of India* (*Countess of Dufferin's Fund*): *Proceedings of the Special Meeting Held at Government House, Calcutta 6th March 1912 at 11 o'clock a.m.*

5. The wording was widely used in the literature of the Dufferin Fund, such as its annual reports.

6. For reasons that remain unclear, Elizabeth Beilby's name is to be found spelled either "Beilby" or "Bielby": see *BMJ* 3 October 1881, 673. At the time of her audience with the queen, "Beilby" is the more normally used version, and it is also how she signed her own name in correspondence; I have accordingly used that version here.

7. *Indian Female Evangelist* VI (October 1881), 145–48; *Jnl. NIA* (1883), 200; *BMJ*, 3 October 1885; *Englishwoman's Review* 14, no. 4 (15 April 1885): 147; *Indian Female Evangelist* 8 (July 1886); Norman Chevers, *Commentary on the Diseases of India* (London, 1886), 713; *BMJ*, 26 April 1890; *London School of Medicine for Women Magazine* 5 (October 1896): 197–202.

8. Anshu Malhotra, "Of Dais and Midwives: 'Middle Class Interventions in the Management of Women's Reproductive Health'—A Study from Colonial Punjab." *Indian Journal of Gender Studies* 10, no. 2 (2003): 229–59.

9. *RA* VIC/MAIN/QVJ/1881: 13 July 1881.

10. The *Indian Female Evangelist* quoted the queen's words as, "WE SHOULD WISH IT GENERALLY KNOWN THAT WE SYMPATHISE WITH EVERY EFFORT MADE TO RELIEVE THE SUFFERING STATE OF THE WOMEN OF INDIA." *Indian Female Evangelist* 6 (October 1881): 145.

11. *RA* PPTO/PP/QV/MAIN/1882/12808, Sir William Muir to Col. Sandwith, 3 February 1882; Interserve: Indian Female Normal School and Instruction Society (IFNSIS) *Minutes* 6 July 1881, Minutes 828–29; ibid., 7 December 1881, Minute 956; E. Beilby, "Zenana Medical Missionaries," *Indian Female Evangelist* 6 (July 1882): 297–302.

12. *RA* VIC/ADDA5/503.

13. *RA* PPTO/PP/QV/MAIN/1882/12808, Muir to Sandwith, 3 February 1882; *RA* PPTO/PP/QV/MAIN/1881/11928, Col. Sandwith to the Duchess of Atholl, 5 July 1881; *Indian Female Evangelist* 6 (October 1881): 147–48.

14. *RA* PPTO/PP/QV/MAIN/1882/12808, Muir to Sandwith, 3 February 1882.

15. Ibid., General Ponsonby to Muir, 26 February 1882; ibid., Muir to Ponsonby, 27 February 1882. The Maharajah had, in fact, sent the queen via Beilby his own portrait, of himself, his three brothers, and a nephew: *RA* PPTO/PP/QV/MAIN/1881/11928, Beilby to Lady Gainsborough, 5 July 1881.

16. *RA* PPTO/PP/QV/MAIN/1882/14808, Queen Victoria's handwritten addendum to Ponsonby to Queen Victoria (QV), 30 November 1882.

17. *PRONI*: D.1071/J/G/7B/3/1 *The Women's Missionary Magazine of the United Presbyterian Church* 8, no. 10 (May 1895): 253; *PRONI*: D.1071 3/C2/5/1–7; *RA* VIC/MAIN/QVJ/1884: 22–25 October 1884.

18. Philip Guedella, *The Queen and Mr. Gladstone, 1880–1898* (London: Hodder and Stoughton, 1933), 249.

19. *RA* VIC/MAIN/M59/14, Hariot Dufferin (HD) to QV, June 1885.

20. The draft prospectus is *RA* VIC/MAIN/M59/17a, enclosure within *RA* VIC/MAIN/M59/17, HD to QV, 7 August [1885]. The printed version is *RA* VIC/MAIN/M/59/18a.

21. *RA* VIC/MAIN/M59/18, HD to QV, 14 August 1885; *RA*: PPTO/PP/QV/1885/2411.

22. *RA* VIC/MAIN/M59/19b. The clipping bears no indication of its provenance. See also *RA* PPTO/PP/QV/MAIN/1885/2411 and *RA* VIC/MAIN/N/43/26.

23. *PRONI*: D.1071.J/G/4A/1; K. A. Knox, *The National Association for Supplying Female Medical Aid to the Women of India* (Calcutta, February 1887).

24. *Times*, 22 August 1887, 24 October 1887.

25. *PRONI*: D.1071.J/G/1A/3, Minutes of the Central Committee of the Countess of Dufferin's Fund: 21 May 1900, letter from H. H. Risley to E. H. Fenn, 28 April 1900.

26. She wrote to Sir Henry Acland in 1898 that medical missions "always seem to me to represent the best form that missionary effort can take, and the most successful, and I should always be glad to see them multiplied." Bodleian Library: Acland MSS d.89/1 HD to HWA, 8 December 1898.

27. *BLAAS*: L/R/5/12, *Reports on Native Newspapers (Bengal) 1886*, 921.

28. Lady Dufferin had proposed appointing a missionary doctor to the new Ripon Hospital. *RA* VIC/MAIN/M59/13, HD to QV, 26 May 1885; *RA* VIC/MAIN/N/43/26, HD to QV, 19 October [1885].

29. *PRONI*: D.1071.J/G/7B1/1-2, *Medical Missions at Home and Abroad* n.s. 2, no. 1 (October 1887): 5.

30. *PRONI*: D.1071.J/G/8/1, H. Cooper to the editor of *Indian Witness*, 15 August 1887.

31. *National Association for Supplying Female Medical Aid to the Women of India: Countess of Dufferin's Fund*: *30th Report of the Madras Branch* (Madras: Government Press, 1916).

32. *PRONI*: D.1071/J/G/3/7.

33. "D. Y.," "A Chat about India (Hints to Those Going to India)," *London School of Medicine for Women Magazine* (17 October 1900): 688–95.

34. *RA* VIC/MAIN/M/60/3a, Shailajanund Ojhah, *An Appeal for the Countess Dufferin Fund* (sic), 7.

35. *BLAAS*: L/R/5/12 *Rpt.Nat.News*. 1886, 266: *Surabhi and Patáká*, 18 February 1886; *RA* VIC/MAIN/M/60/3 HD to QV, 27 January 1886.

36. *RA* VIC/MAIN/M/60/3a, Ojbah, *Appeal,* 10.

37. *BLAAS*: L/R/5/11 *Rpt.Nat.News*. 1885, 1477: *Ananda Bazar Patrika*, 24 August 1885; ibid., 1151: *Praja Bandhu*, 4 September 1885.

38. Ibid., 1104: *Samvád Prabhákar*, 22 August 1885.

39. *BLAAS*: L/R/5/7 *Rpt.Nat.News*. 1881: *Dacca Prakash*, 1 May 1881; L/R/5/12 *Rpt.Nat.News*. 1886, 1196–7: *Sanjivani*, 30 October 1886.

40. *BLAAS*: L/R/5/12 *Rpt.Nat.News*. 1886, 204: *Bharát Mihir*, 4 February 1886.

41. *BLAAS*: L/R/5/16 *Rpt.Nat.News*. 1890, 1051: *Dainik-o-Samáchar Chandriká*, 17 November 1890; L/R/5/17 *Rpt.Nat.News*. 1891, 1003: *Navayuga*, 10 September 1891; ibid., 226: *Sanjivani*, 1 March 1890.

42. Marchioness of Dufferin and Ava, *Our Viceregal Life in India: Selections from My Journal, 1884–1888*, 2 vols. (London: John Murray, 1889).

43. *BLAAS*: L/R/5/11 *Rpt.Nat.News*. 1885, 1033: *Arya Darfan*, 7 August 1885; ibid., 1038: *Bhárat Basi*, 8 August 1885; L/R/5/11 *Rpt.Nat.News*. 1885, 653: *Bhárat Mihir*, 6 August 1885.

44. This caused a procedural dilemma in 1875 when the Prince of Wales visited India. See *RA* VIC/MAIN/Z/468/10 Lord Northbrooke to Lord Salisbury, 29 April 1875.

45. *BLAAS*: L/R/5/11 *Rpt.Nat.News*. 1885, 1105: *Sádhárani*, 23 August 1885.

46. Ibid., 1105: *Sádhárani*, 23 August 1885, 1263–4: *Sádhárani*, 27 September 1885.

47. *BLAAS*: L/R/5/14 *Rpt.Nat.News*. 1888, 227: *Dacca Gazette*, 20 February 1888.

48. Ibid., 426: *Education Gazette*, 13 April 1888.

49. *PRONI*: D.1071/J/G/6/2.

50. *PRONI*: D.1071/J/G/6/2.

51. *PRONI*: D.1071/J/G/6/2.

52. *PRONI*: D.1071/J/G/6/2.

53. Marchioness of Dufferin and Ava, "The Women of India," *The Nineteenth Century*, vol. 29 (January–June 1891), 359–66.

54. *PRONI*: D.1071/J/G/6/2.

55. Tanika Sarkar, "Nationalist Iconography: Image of Women in Nineteenth-Century Bengali Literature," *Economic and Political Weekly*, 21 November 1987, 2011–15.

56. *BLAAS*: L/R/5/11 *Rpt.Nat.News*. 1885, 1477: *Dacca Prakash*, 6 December 1885.

57. Ibid., 1477: *Bheri*, 27 November 1885.

58. *BLAAS*: L/R/5/14 *Rpt.Nat.News*. 1888, 1063: *Sanjivani*, 13 October 1888.

59. *PRONI*: D.1071.J/G/3/3 K. Ganguli to Secretary to Central Committee of the Dufferin Fund, 3 December 1888.

60. *BLAAS*: L/R/5/16 *Rpt.Nat.News*. 1890, 1051: *Dainik-o-Samáchar Chandriká*, 17 November 1890; L/R/5/17 *Rpt.Nat.News*. 1891, 241: *Dainik-o-Samáchar Chandriká*, 17 February 1891.

61. *BLAAS*: L/R/5/13 *Rpt.Nat.News*. 1887, 521–22: *Sanjivani*, 14 May 1887; L/R/5/16 *Rpt.Nat.News*. 1890, 225:*Sanjivani*, 1 March 1890.

62. Lal, "Politics of Gender and Medicine," 37.

63. *Pioneer*, 18 September 1896.

64. *BLAAS*: L/R/5/15 *Rpt.Nat.News*. 1889, 265: *Prajá Bandhu*, 22 March 1889; ibid., 266: *Sanjivani*, 23 March 1889.

65. *BLAAS*: L/R/5/14 *Rpt.Nat.News*. 1888, 425: *Surabhi and Pataka*, 12 April 1888.

66. *BLAAS*: L/R/5/13 *Rpt.Nat.News*. 1887, 143: *Samaya*, 28 January 1887.

67. Lal, "Politics of Gender and Medicine," 65. European women doctors objected to the practice but were not able to reverse it; when the Dufferin Fund became the basis for the new Women's Medical Service for India in 1913, male supervision was written into its regulations. *BLAAS*: P/V 492 *Proceedings of the Special Meeting*, 6 March 1912; *PRONI*: D.1071 J/G/4A/5 *Women's Medical Service for India: General Rules and Regulations*.

Chapter Seven

Educating Lady Doctors in Colonial Burma

Missionaries, the Lady Dufferin Hospital, and the Local Government in the Making of Burmese Medical Women

Atsuko Naono

Various scholars have examined white lady missionaries as key agents of the imperial enterprise, shouldering a female version of "white man's burden" for their colonized female "sisters."[1] This research has directed particular attention to these missionaries' peculiar status, ideas, and agendas that determined the colonial gendered spheres, the feminine sphere characterized by domesticity, childbirth and rearing, and women's health. The impact on colonized women was profound; these lady missionaries undertook campaigns to transform indigenous women according to their model into "good mothers and wives" by educating them in hygiene, sanitation, nutrition, and maternity.[2] In British India, there were also nongovernmental associations concerned with the health of the female indigenous population of the empire. Among the most important was the Lady Dufferin Fund that became a major force in reaffirming the gendered spheres of medical space introduced by earlier generations of the lady missionary doctors.

In India, Lal identifies the ideological and political importance of gender and health issues to colonial rule, which drew legitimation from the perception of indigenous backwardness in both areas. Social reform campaigns were, thus, an important feature of the colonial period.[3] Lady Dufferin, wife of the viceroy of India, led one such program, the National Association for Supplying Female Medical Aid to the Women of India. This association campaigned to provide medical aid and education to the women of India often with the simple assertion that Indian women would not consult with male physicians.[4] The Dufferin Fund effort to foster the growth of Indian lady doctors had limited success partly because it could not draw sufficient numbers of female students from among upper-class Hindu and Muslim families.[5] In addition to the limitations imposed by *purdah*, there were also difficulties presented by the low female literacy rate and poor general education that contributed to the slow pace of raising Indian medical women. Although the limitations of purdah did not exist among the indigenous population in colonial Burma, and Burmese women reportedly enjoyed independence and relative freedom in their social activities, the emergence of medical women there also took considerable time.

Health practices related to maternity provide a useful focus for this chapter, for almost no health issue was as neglected by indigenous doctors as childbirth and here the impact of Western medicine on indigenous medical practices was arguably most dramatic. It is, perhaps, for this reason that research on the history of women's health in colonial India and elsewhere in Southeast Asia has focused on this subject.[6] In this chapter, I will examine the development of medical women in Burma focusing on the practices of local midwives called *wan zwe* (literally, "pulling the womb" in Burmese) targeted by medical missionaries as well as by the Lady Dufferin Fund. I will also explore the ways in which the category of "Burmese midwifery" was constructed through the interaction of Baptist missionary lady doctors, the Lady Dufferin Hospital, and the local government, an intersection that played a crucial role in influencing the development of indigenous medical women in the province of Burma in British India. Lastly, I will examine how the local population of Burma treated the newly qualified indigenous medical women who practiced Western midwifery and obstetrics in opposition to the local *wan zwe*.

The Lady Dufferin Fund frequently criticized Indian local practices of midwifery by *dais*, hereditary midwives who belonged to lower-caste families, in legitimating their campaign to train Indian midwives and improve medical care for Indian women. In Burma, the colonial medical officers as well as missionary doctors made similar attacks toward indigenous midwives. The peculiarities of the Burmese version of midwife, the *wan zwe*, and especially of her "barbaric" practices, were frequently reported by numerous early Western medical observers. Lady Dufferin herself described the practices of the *wan zwe* as "especially barbarous," reporting its practice using sensational words such as the mother being "nearly baked and dried up."[7] Many medical men argued the imminent necessity to eradicate the *wan zwe*. For example, C. C. Little, an inspector-general of Civil Hospitals, Burma, stated, "Let us trust, of ultimately ousting altogether from the field the midwives of the old school with their ignorant and brutal methods."[8] British colonial medical authorities as well as Christian missionaries viewed midwifery and nursing to be the main domains in which indigenous women could play a major role. When the Countess Dufferin hospital was opened in Rangoon in 1887, the school for nursing and midwifery opened together with the hospital seeking to provide medical treatments to women and children. The improvement of midwifery and nursing seems to have been one of the most serious issues to overcome in view of the high rates of infant mortality as well as maternity deaths among the indigenous population in the colony. Earlier literature has focused on poor infant diets as the main factor in the high rate of child deaths in Burma. For example, Richell suggests that the vitamin-poor diet of chewed rice mothers gave their children and the longer lactating period, were the major reasons for high infant mortality.[9] However, despite the volume of colonial accounts of health in Burma, there has been little examination of the *wan zwe* practices that were in fact the major determinant of maternity and infant deaths.

Much of the story of the emergence of the categories of Burmese medicine and Burmese midwifery were shaped by the intersection of the trajectory of the expansion of the British East India Company, on the one hand, and the unconscious division of labor between the British and American Missionary Societies on the other. British missionaries, for example, first entered South Asia through the East India Company lands in the early nineteenth century before the company had yet expanded into Burma. At the same time, American Baptist Missionaries had selected a yet unconquered Burma as the first Baptist mission anywhere in the world. As the Company and then the British government annexed parts of Burma over the next few decades, they also incorporated American Baptist Missions that had already established a dominant missionary position.

American Baptist missionaries played a determining role in categorizing the culture of Burmese midwifery and related practices through daily interaction with the local population. The main force in these efforts were white lady doctors who came to Burma with a perspective of health, medicine, and home that isolated medical practices related to women's and children's health within a sphere of activity best handled by women.[10] Although there were occasional male commentators, they usually based their descriptions on information provided by lady doctors or in their association with the women. The prime example is Dr. T. F. Pedley, a Rangoon-based, internationally known general practitioner and author of articles on Burmese midwifery, who was heavily involved with the female doctors at work at the Dufferin hospital; Dr. Pedley was a member of the management committee as a honorary physician as well as independent lady missionary doctors, such as Dr. May Fowler-Thompson.

These doctors collectively have left us with a rich archive of material through which to investigate the encounter between Western medical practitioner and Burmese patient in the late nineteenth century and in doing so they shed light on the intellectual roots of the emergence of Burmese practitioners of Western obstetrical medicine from the early decades of the twentieth century. Dr. Fowler-Thompson has been more broadly important in this article not so much for the data mobilized, but for providing a "feel" for the period and the encounter. She is significant in understanding and putting the engagement between lady missionary doctors and the Burmese medical practices into a daily context in large part because she appears to be the only doctor, male or female, who has left a diary of their medical practice in Burma in the late nineteenth century. The diary covers in detail the daily highlights of her encounter with Burmese patients and their reactions to Western medical practices. Sometimes humorous, and sometimes horrific, the anecdotes reveal the frustrations that the white lady doctor and the Burmese patients had regarding each other and the cultural difference between them. For our purposes here, however, it was mainly Dr. Fowler-Thompson's associates, Dr. Pedley and Dr. Douglass, who contributed most to the discourse of Burmese midwifery and their practice and understanding, revealed in their published research findings and observations in medical journals of the day and on the pages of Douglass's doctoral thesis, that are the most important focus of our attention here.

Some details about the childbirth process, such as those related to the preparation of the laboring room, merely exorcized the practice. The delivery of the baby usually takes place in confinement in the upper room of the house on the stills and bamboo floors, separated from other rooms "by hanging a thick curtain or screen across it."[11] Further, since the Burmese believed that the burning smell of oil and fat from cooking cause illness and death, the laboring room was carefully shut air tight as much as possible so that the mother is not exposed to those smells. In this airtight room, they boiled the water. There were several female attendants, mostly the mother's family and relatives besides the *wan zwe*.

Christian missionary doctors and their government associates, such as Dr. Pedley, however, were horrified by the pressures put on the woman's body throughout the entire process of childbirth. This began with the onset of labor and the *wan zwe*'s forceful and violent pushing of the mother's abdomen. As Douglass explained:

> A Burman woman . . . is laid on a mat on the bamboo floor, and without the least idea of position or presentation, with every pain is subjected to such pressure as the midwife may think the case demands, in order to press the child downward. As it descends, a piece of cloth is bound tightly about the mother to prevent its retrieving to its former position. If kneading the mother with the hands does not produce the desired effect, the midwife as her assistant she herself by holding on to some object, places one part above the child, and with heel and toe movements, tries to press the child down. Should this means fail, then other methods are employed. The most common is to take a bamboo yoke such as is used by the coolies, and watermen in carrying their burdens, and

> lying it across the mother above the child, two persons sit, one on either end of the bamboo, and press the child steadily down. This is constantly done in cases of abnormal position and almost always end in rupturing the uterus, and often in killing both mother and child.[12]

Pedley directed more extensive attention to the use of band or cloth tightly tied around the mother's body until the ejection of the placenta. The main purpose of this band was not, as might be supposed, to compress the uterus or restrict hemorrhage after birth. Instead, because it was tied above the umbilicus, it was clearly intended solely to prevent the possibility of the placenta and the uterus rising up into the chest cavity. Further, at the point when the baby's head pressed the perineum, the *wan zwe* would have other attending women keep continuous pressure on the abdomen and "if it be a first child [the *wan zwe*] makes a tear in the perineum with her thumb-nail, which is allowed to grow sharp and long for this purpose." After the child was extracted, the cord was cut, and they continued to put pressure on the abdomen to extract the placenta. The *wan zwe*'s hand was employed to drag it out in the case that the extraction does not go smoothly. After the child was born there was also an overemphasis on the recovery of normal positioning of the abdomen of the mothers from their "swollen external genitals." In Pedley's view, too much pressure was put on to the uterus, sometimes with the foot. This practice was linked with the Burmese notion of the body and the *wan zwes* curiously believed that the joints were relaxed after delivery and needed to be restored, sometimes by stamping upon them.[13]

The use of excessive force was also, we are told, due to the fear of the bad spirit, nats, which was of greater concern than the health of the mother or the child. It was for this reason that the birthing process was marked by a special ceremony that began as soon as the newborn baby was washed.

> The grandmother or nearest female relative on the mother's side, shoves it along the floor, saying, "Here witches came and take it, Here devils came and eat it." The idea is to propitiate all the spirits that might otherwise work evil to the child. But when as is often the case, the infant is shocked and convultious, the whole house is in an uproar, saying "The nats have caught it," and at once offerings of all sorts are made to the spirits, to corks them not of the child. If the babe dies, its little body is not allowed to remain in the house over night, because if it did, the woman would not have another child.[14]

Even then, the Burmese mother's ordeal was not over. Instead of resting, the mother was quickly washed, the entire body rubbed with turmeric, and her vulva plastered with saffron. Then, the mother was immediately held in confinement and subjected to extreme heating and cooling for the following ten days. According to Douglass, the mother was immediately placed next to a big fire with her body being wrapped in a thick woolen curtain. The smoke from this fireplace irritated the conjunctiva of the mother and of her child and was a major source for distress.[15] Then, "Hot bricks are placed around the abdomen to increase the flow, the object being to cleanse the system from impurities."[16] She was not allowed to take cold food or drink and everything was prepared piping hot with black pepper. The diet mainly consisted of salt fish and rice.[17] Further, the mother had to "sit over hot coals upon where powdered turmeric has been thrown."[18] The Burmese were said to believe that "the heat . . . penetrates to the internal parts and heals them."[19] The peak of heating came on the eighth and ninth day with the mother's entire body from head to toe wrapped with thick blankets. Her bed was surrounded with heavy curtains while she was exposed to a "severe vapor-bath" produced by a "large supply of hot bricks" until she could sweat freely.[20] Then, on the tenth day of this extreme heating, an extreme cooling process began with "cold water drawn fresh from the well poured over head and all."[21] As Douglass' native assistant, Ma Bain, who persevered through this ordeal, admitted, "this was worse than the agony of giving birth to the child."[22]

As with other contests between Burmese and Western medicine, the nefarious practices of indigenous medicine were identified with a particular group of practitioners and the latter were demonized. In this case, Burmese midwives were viewed as the purveyors of death and had to be stopped, in part because they appeared to retain the loyalty of most Burmese patients in the face of the "undeniable truth" of Western medicine. According to Pedley, *wan zwe*, lacking in hygienic and anatomical knowledge and frequently "decrepit hags, half blind with age, were also

> generally of the poorest and lowest class, often much advanced in years, whose right to practice is chiefly grounded on the fact that they have been mothers and grandmothers of many. None of them have—any more than the doctors—the slightest acquaintance with scientific midwifery.[23]

What bothered Western doctors most was the authority with which *wan zwes* were held by the Burmese in matters of childbirth, and this authority drew party upon the esteem with which older, knowledgeable members of society were held in Burmese culture. As Pedley complained, "The more aged, the more boldly and obstinately they adhere to what they consider the proper method of procedure, and the more highly are they respected. Of course, new methods, or any kind of innovation or interference, are stubbornly resisted."[24]

The last point is most relevant here, for the *wan zwes*, just as was the case with inoculators in the struggle against smallpox,[25] were viewed as the main reason for the slow pace of the introduction of Western obstetrical medicine among the Burmese. This was evidenced by the fact that it was the Burmese patients who put up a shield of protection around the Burmese midwives.

Douglass's 1882 doctoral thesis provides several examples from her own experiences in Rangoon. In one case, a Christian missionary nurse, for example, tried to stop four of these *wan zwe* cases carried out near their mission house in Moulmein, but was powerless to prevent the relatives from following the advice of the heathen midwife. In another case, Mr. Wilkes, a druggist in Moulmein, was so upset about *wan zwe* practices that he obtained permission for a postmortem examination of the cadaver of the dead mother along with an arrest warrant for the *wan zwe*. This postmortem examination concluded,

> The uterus had been ruptured from side to side, the body of the child forced into the cavity of the bowels, and the child's head separated from the body by the pressure which had been used.[26]

To complement their disparagement, the *wan zwes* were attributed with the basest of motives—money and the worst of outcomes. As Pedley stressed, while midwives in Madras limited their fee to "a miserable pittance of a few pence," midwives in Burma demanded varying sums from five rupees to thirty or forty rupees, a small fortune by contrast. For this high price, tetanus was a common result and the cause of death for many of the Burmese mothers, a uniquely Burmese phenomenon caused by midwives and their "violent pressure to a greater or less extent . . . used for several hours."[27]

Nevertheless, reasons were given for why greater success might be experienced here than on the subcontinent. Most importantly, unlike the case with the Indian *dais*, Western doctors here did not have to contend with the limitations of caste and female seclusion. As Pedley commented,

> The Burmah caste, with its social rules and restriction, is unknown, and unlike the women of India, Burmese women freely accept the aid of Europeans or their own male physicians.[28]

Further, Burmese willingly accepted Western medical aid as a last resort, unable to consult their own doctors for religious reasons. As Dr. MacDonald, one of the Western physicians, observed,

> According to their religious belief, when a woman dies in childbed she is considered unclean, consequently cannot enter into the state of *neiban*, or total annihilation (the Heaven of the Burmese), so that there is an inducement to seek the aid of Europeans whom they know by experience to be capable of doing what they cannot do themselves, especially when their own nostrums fail in affording relief.[29]

While white lady doctors viewed colonial India's midwifery and childbirth as highly gendered practices, those of the Burmese were viewed as rather culturally determined and less gender specific, but still dangerous practices.

Medical missionaries were the initial driving force in the training of indigenous women in nursing and midwifery. With the development of modern medicine, the Christian medical missionary became more active worldwide, the motivation being to gain popularity and trust among indigenous populations. In 1853, for example, the Baptist Missionary Convention had approved the employment of medical work as a means of evangelization.[30] Before this, there were already several Christian missionaries engaged in medical work in Burma. The American Baptist Mission was one of the first contingents to arrive in Burma in the early nineteenth century and it commenced its medical work there in the 1820s. British medical missionaries mainly focused on the subcontinent, leaving Lower Burma, the main area of British Burma until the Third Anglo-Burmese War in 1885, to American missionary efforts.

An unusual feature of missionary medical work in Lower Burma was the predominance of female doctors. Those of the Woman's American Baptist Foreign Mission Society dominated the medical work in Lower Burma from the 1880s. Dr. Ellen Mitchell, the first woman missionary doctor in Burma, opened her work in Moulmein at the age of fifty and dedicated the last twenty-two years of her life to the medical work in Lower Burma.[31] Mitchell arrived with a trained nurse named Miss A. M. Barkley. They were so enthusiastic about teaching that Mitchell began the course on hygiene from the first year and Barkley began her nursing course immediately as well.[32] One of the difficulties of initial medical education was in large part derived from Burma's diverse ethnic and linguistic communities, each with their own medical traditions and practices, leading Mitchell to complain of having to contend with "over a thousand treatments among sixteen nationalities" in one year.[33] It does not seem that Mitchell's medical education was massively successful during her life. Due to the high demand of nurses, Barkley was transferred soon after to Zigon, near Prome in Lower Burma. In her place, Mitchell received a new associate, a Burmese male physician named Dr. Shaw Lu, who received his medical education at the American Baptist Bucknell College. In order to make their medicine attractive among the local population, they put their fellow Burmese preacher, Ko Yan Gin, in charge of selling simple medicine alongside the scripture he distributed at the local bazaar to the people from "their jungle homes."[34] This medical missionary work in Moulmein was halted with Mitchell's death in 1901 until it revived again in 1917 with the construction of the Ellen Mitchell Memorial Hospital for women and children with money raised by the local Mon community[35] and it included a nursing school led by American nurses.[36]

Meanwhile, the lady doctors at the Dufferin Hospital were also making headway in educating indigenous medical women in Rangoon. The Dufferin Hospital in Rangoon was opened in a large rented bungalow in 1887 after failing to make the female wards of the Rangoon Hospital a maternity hospital.[37] As in India, even though it was supposed to be a private hospital, it was actually funded by both the local government and the Municipal Committee of Rangoon with grants of about 4,000 rupees annually each.

Dr. Maria Douglass from the American Baptist Missionary was recruited as the first resident medical officer and superintendent. Dr. Maria C. Douglass received medical training in America and returned to Burma in 1882 after marrying to Rev. J. D. Douglass, the first Baptist missionary to Karens at Bassein, Douglass.[38] Douglass graduated from the Woman's Medical College of Pennsylvania (WMCP) in 1882 and she wrote a thesis titled: "The Medical Practice and Obstetrics of the Burmese and Karens." This thesis, archived in Drexel University College of Medicine, has the long history of female medical education of WMCP. Many female graduates from the WMCP provided their medical work as medical missionaries. Along with Dr. Maria Douglass, Brigade-Surgeon Griffith was also appointed as consulting medical officer and Dr. Pedley, health officer of Rangoon, served as honorary secretary of the hospital.[39]

The government's annual reports on hospitals in the colony for 1902 called the Dufferin Hospital in Rangoon "the only institution of the exclusive use of females, combining a maternity and lying-in-hospital with the treatment of general diseases of women and children and providing for the training of nurses and midwives."[40] Up until 1898, the development of the Dufferin Hospital appeared successful as it trained at least one hundred women in midwifery and nursing "acquainted with the Burmese language."[41] They proudly reported that all of these women were serving in various parts of the province. However, about this time, the Dufferin Hospital actually began to get involved in serious friction with the local government. There emerged quite a bitter struggle for control over the Dufferin Hospital and it seriously affected the production of indigenous midwives and nurses. Problems emerged between Sir Frederic Fryer, the lieutenant governor of Burma, and the Committee of the Dufferin Hospital in Rangoon when the committee refused to endorse Fryer's wishes to appoint a particular lady doctor as superintendent and resident doctor of the Dufferin Hospital. The Committee of the Dufferin Hospital viewed this candidate as being inappropriate for the post since she lacked Burmese language skills, which the committee saw as one of the most important qualifications for the training of native women. In retaliation, Fryer threatened the committee with the withdrawal of both grants from the government and the Municipality of Rangoon from the hospital. Finally, the committee gave in. Flushed with this victory, Fryer made a further demand, that the committee allow this lady doctor to engage in private practice as well her hospital duties, even though this would contradict the Dufferin Hospital's policies. The committee members and local Rangoon subscribers, infuriated with Fryer's new demand, renewed their opposition to the governor, this time more vigorously.[42] Reportedly, Fryer achieved his controversial second wish by abusing his power and authority. Fryer sent supporters to attend the next committee meeting and vote in his favor despite not being elected members of the committee. He even excluded reporters for the local newspapers from attending this meeting. The high-handed manner with which the lieutenant governor executed his plan was understandably treated negatively by the press, which reports,

> Sir. F. Fryer is evidently determined to carry out his own views concerning the management of the hospital without reference to the wishes of the local subscribers, and the result of all this strife must inevitably be damaging to the work of a most admirable charity.[43]

The bitter feeling this friction left must have been considerable. Lord George Hamilton, secretary of state for India, in his letter to Sir Hugh Barnes, Fryer's successor as lieutenant governor of Burma, states, "The result certainly has been, I think, very considerably to damage the efficacy of the institution, and apparently to divert it from the original object for which funds were solicited."[44] Hamilton asked Barnes to rectify the deteriorated relationship between the government and the committee in order to "get the civil population to work with you in maintaining the hospital."[45]

The Dufferin Hospital was not the only formalized training institute for Burmese women doctors to emerge in this period. In Moulmein and Bassein, other hospitals were active as well. At Bassein, Dr. May Fowler-Thompson[46] was another American Baptist medical missionary as well as the president of the Burma branch of Women's Christian Temperance Union (WCTU). Dr. Fowler-Thompson was appointed to serve in mission schools as well as Carpenter Memorial Hospital in Bassein[47] from 1892 and in Rangoon from 1893. While in Bassein, she began her teaching by providing a nurses' training class to local seventh standard schoolgirls.[48]

The impact of Western medical training was intended to be across classes. For example, the Dufferin Hospital sought to make training affordable to poorer Burmese women with the award of six scholarships and a monthly stipend of ten rupees in 1887.[49] At the same time, it benefited from the recruitment of an elite classmate for these women, the Myingoondine princess, a granddaughter of King Mindon of the last Burmese dynasty. She had medical training in Rangoon "with the view of qualifying herself to practice among her Burmese fellow-countrywomen."[50]

Despite early progress, recruitment declined in the following decade. This was most likely due to the Dufferin Fund's major friction with the local government as discussed above. In 1900, for example, there were twenty-four pupil midwives who underwent a midwifery course and training in sick nursing.[51] However, in 1901, there were only twelve pupil midwives and the number further dropped to eight in 1902.[52] As the number of prospective indigenous medical women dropped, King, an inspector general of Civil Hospitals, Burma, complaining, "It was found hopeless to secure female hospital assistants," the government became concerned. By 1906, it began undertaking serious efforts to entice the indigenous female population to the midwifery training, including the creation of two scholarships for "partially trained [Burmese] women in Madras."[53]

The government viewed the lack of employment opportunities for these indigenous medical women to be the major reason for the unpopularity of their scheme. D. Shearme, Secretary to the Government of Burma, stated,

> A scheme has been prepared in consultation with the committee whereby a training will be given in this hospital to Burmese and Karen women in midwifery, and employment has been guaranteed under Municipal or District Cess Funds for over twenty of these women when trained.[54]

The government responded by applying measures in Burma that had been successful on the subcontinent. It adopted the "Result-System Midwives" scheme, which was successful in Madras Presidency. In sanctioning this scheme, the government granted a large amount of funding for the building of quarters for the midwifery training courses as well as the annual grants to the ten candidates.[55] Although the government issued a self-congratulatory report on the success of the "Result-System midwives," they have only ten students annually and even then, already in 1910, they were unable to completely fill the ten positions.[56]

While the Dufferin Hospital was having difficulty in increasing the number of female students, the government decided to begin their own government medical school in 1907 that included native female students such as Ma Nallie Pathie, the first female medical student from the Baptist Karen Mission, in this new medical school. However, they clearly had some difficulty in attracting a significant number of female students. While the number of male students increased steadily from fourteen in 1907 to 209 in 1921, the number of female students remained quite low (see table 7.1).

Although the trajectory of women's medical training in Burma had been set by female medical missionaries and the Dufferin's Hospital to be within the female sphere of the medical activity, the institutional ethos of the Dufferin Hospital, as a quasi-government institution, was still dominated by what

Table 7.1. Number of students taught at the Government Medical School at Rangoon

Year	Male	Female	Total
1907	14	1	15
1908	12	1	13
1909	32	3	35
1910	37	6	43
1911	44	4	48
1912	56	6	62
1913	50	6	56
1914	56	5	61
1915	68	7	75
1916	N. A.	N. A.	100
1917	107	7	114
1918	140	7	147
1919	158	7	165
1920	190	7	197
1921	209	12	221

From *Report on the Working of the Government Medical School, Rangoon*, for various years 1907–1922 (Rangoon: Office of the Superintendent, Government Printing, Burma)

Lal refers to as an "imperial gender ideology." The goals of the Lady Dufferin Fund had all along been implicitly directed at eventually having men take over the management of the hospitals.[57]

There were thus increasing efforts by some government medical men to bring those activities within the male sphere of the medical profession as well. These efforts began slowly and were insidious. At this new medical school, male medical students began undertaking a midwifery course, which was included only in the final year until 1912, but expanded into both the third and the fourth years from 1913 onward. In addition, after passing the examination, male students were sent to the Government Maternity Hospital in Madras for practical training for midwifery for three months while female students were sent to receive the same training at the Dufferin Hospital in Rangoon. The cost of this practical midwifery training at Madras put extra financial pressure on the tight budgets of the hospital and it was also inconvenient to the male students as well.[58] Despite these disadvantages, the government continued sending male medical students to Madras. Even when it came to nursing, the medical establishment sometimes preferred recruiting men rather than taking the trouble to locate female staff. In one case, the government approved a suggestion, made by Mergui civil surgeon Dr. Evans, to utilize the indigenous male compounders to be trained in technical nursing and employ them as "ward-assistants."[59] These attempts to push indigenous male medical students to undertake midwifery and nursing might have been encouraged by the medical establishment on the basis of the simple observation that there was no limitation of female seclusion in Burma comparable to that in India.

Despite these efforts to redefine women's medicine as a male medical practice, by the end of the colonial period, midwifery and obstetrics remained in a female medical domain conducted exclusively by lady doctors. The colonial medical establishment does not appear to provide any answers as to why, despite extensive efforts to train native males to undertake these practical trainings, they remained the almost exclusive preserve of female medical doctors. This could be due to several reasons; first, it could be because despite the efforts to train males in midwifery, the missionary lady doctor efforts from the late nineteenth century had been successful in creating the permanent intellectual category of midwifery and obstetrics as women's medicine. As a result, Burmese males, although given training in midwifery, opted for medical activities after graduation that had not been so clearly defined as within the female sphere. Second, related to the first reason, midwifery and obstetrics probably remained at the bottom of the status hierarchy of medical practices in Burma, and Burmese lady doctors may have been directed to those activities while being excluded from other medical fields. In either or both cases, divisions that had been created by medical missionaries outside of the government medical establishment had ultimately shaped government medicine by the end of the colonial period. Third, another possibility is that missionary lady doctors had also been successful in infusing the practice of women's medicine with some of their missionizing zeal, giving new generations of native lady doctors a real sense of purpose and meaning in treating their female compatriots.

Lastly, one of the most important questions would be the impact of indigenous medical women regarding the local population's responses toward Western medicine. It is difficult to say this was absolute certainty as there are few available indigenous sources to prove this. However, we have several sources such as newspaper articles and the proceedings of the legislative council that shed some light on the indigenous reaction to the emergence of Western-trained medical women in Burma.

It appears that some parts of Burma, especially areas with a strong Christian presence, were willing to support and appreciate the work of midwives with a Western medical education. In Sagaing, for example, when the civil hospital opened there in 1915, it had a "well-equipped" maternity ward. It was the work of the native lady medical officer and nurse, Ma Thet Su, however, that made the maternity ward popular among the local population, having forty-five admissions within just over half a year. As the local newspaper commented on the positive response from the local population, "The splendid result would not have been possible without the cooperation of the Burmese ladies and elders of Sagaing generally, who have been instrumental in preaching the benefits of the maternity ward and inducing patients to attend."[60] There were also a number of charitable local organizations that became quite active in promoting the training of midwives and nurses so that they could aid childbirth among indigenous mothers in Burma. For example, the Society for the Prevention of Infantile Mortality was established in 1906 with Burmese leadership. This organization was successful, expanding all over Burma and establishing local branches, enjoying both official and private support.[61] The Burma branch of the Red Cross Society later took over its activities and enthusiastically continued its health propaganda activities in educating mothers and aiding the training of midwives.[62]

However, in the many areas of Burma where Christian influence was less pronounced, such as Mandalay, the local population still resisted Western medicine. In 1920, it was reported that the Burmese *wan zwe* were still more popular among the local population there than were Western-trained midwives. Among 5,550 births registered in Mandalay, only 950 resorted to the western-trained midwives and the remaining 4,600 still chose the *wan zwe* to attend in labor even though the rates of infantile deaths and the mothers' deaths in childbirth were much higher than those attended by qualified midwives.[63] Concerned with the very high infantile mortality caused by the unpopularity of Western-trained midwives on the one hand and the resilient popularity of the *wan zwe* on the other, some members of the legislative council proposed some legal remedies. In 1920, Dr. N. N. Parakh requested that the council put forward a bill for the registration of midwives and nurses, which prohibited the unlicensed practices carried out by the *wan zwe*. However, some members doubted the practicality of the proposed bill due to the insufficient numbers of qualified midwives and nurses to cope with the increased demand that would ensue from the unavailability of the *wan zwe*. Further, there was also a fear that such a drastic change would encourage strong resistance from the local *wan zwe* and might nullify the possibility of any legal measure working. As Mr. Brander expressed, "[It] should not excite any opposition on the part of those who may fear that their means of livelihood are being withdrawn."[64] In the end, the Burma Nurses and Midwives Act was passed in 1922, but it remained largely inactive for at least a decade.[65] The dependency of the local mothers, especially in rural areas, upon the *wan zwe* continued at least up to the close of the war.[66]

This does not mean that there were no prominent indigenous lady doctors trained in Western medicine in colonial Burma. Dr. Ma Saw Sa, for example, received her medical training in the Calcutta Medical School and the University of Dublin and became physician-in-charge and superintendent of the

Dufferin Hospital in Rangoon from 1914 to 1921.[67] In her last year at the Dufferin Hospital, she compiled a medical text on midwifery in Burmese.[68] As another prominent example, Ma H'La Yin was a Mon nurse who received a full two-year course of nurse's training at the Missouri Baptist Sanitarium in the United States, and served at the Ellen Mitchell Hospital at Moulmein from 1921.[69] These two figures are retrospectively viewed as Burmese medical women pioneers now, although many others quickly followed their heels. That this would happen was partly ensured by colonial political reforms, for in 1923, Burma gained limited self-rule (diarchy) and the transfer of the educational and health responsibilities of the government to Burmese ministers, while the civil service began to introduce Burmanization. This meant in part that the transition in leadership in Western medicine occurred before and not after the high-pitch of nationalist efforts and the medical activities in the colony were thus not seen as essentially colonial. Instead, they were depoliticized and accepted as medicine practiced as much by the Burmese as by anyone else. As for the Dufferin Hospital, it continued to promote female medical education in the country for the remainder of colonial rule and after the country's independence in 1948. Indeed, the wife of national father General Aung San was a nurse herself trained at the hospital. In its new Burmese form, nationalized and renamed the Central Women's Hospital, it occupied the strategic centre of successful Burmese efforts to replace autonomous *wan zwe* with trained nurses.

The medical education of indigenous women in colonial Burma developed at the intersection of the efforts of the American women medical missionaries, the Lady Dufferin Fund, and the local government. Although midwifery and obstetrics mostly remained in the domain of lady doctors in the end, the local government's chief male authority, the governor, who highhandedly obtained control over the Dufferin Hospital, played a major role in deterring the Dufferin Hospital's campaign to train indigenous women in midwifery and nursing. In addition, the medical women's dominant position in midwifery and childbirth was often shaken by the colonial government's medical establishment which made vigorous attempts to furnish their medical men with training in midwifery practices. This attempt should have been easier because pre-colonial "Burmese midwifery" was not defined in gendered and caste-specific ways, such as the practices of the *dais* in the subcontinent. Why women remained dominant in women's medicine and obstetrics in Burma was largely due to the impact of the lady missionary doctors. We also should not forget the historical contingency of how "Burmese midwifery" was defined. Through their diaries, reports, and other writings, lady missionary doctors and others associated with the Dufferin Hospital produced a discourse on "Burmese midwifery" that emphasized the horrific, unscientific, and dangerous practices they encountered. The American Baptist Missionaries, who were already actively engaged in medical training in

Burma when the British arrived, would, under British rule, unconsciously preserve the category of "Burmese midwifery," preventing its absorption by another evolving category of indigenous medical practice being developed by British medical men and women whose gaze was centered more on the subcontinent, the rubric of "Indian medicine." This unique circumstance, thus, played an important role in the emergence of indigenous medical women and obstetrical and midwifery practice in Burma.

NOTES

1. Antoinette Burton, "Contesting the Zenana: The Mission to Make 'Lady Doctors for India,' 1874–1885," *Journal of British Studies* 35 (1996): 368–97; Jane Haggis, "Ironies of Emancipation: Changing Configurations of 'Women's Work' in the 'Mission of Sisterhood' to Indian Women," *Feminist Review* 65 (Summer 2000): 108–26.
2. Chie Ikeya, "Scientific and Hygienic Housewife-and-Mother: Education, Consumption and the Discourse of Domesticity," *Journal of Burma Studies* 14 (2010): 65–69; Margaret Jolly, "To Save the Girls for Brighter and Better Lives," *Journal of Pacific History* 26, no. 1 (1991): 27–48.
3. Maneesha Lal, "The Politics of Gender and Medicine in Colonial India: The Countess of Dufferin's Fund, 1885–1888," *Bulletin of the History of Medicine* 68, no. 1 (Spring 1994): 30, 35.
4. Though Lal examines that this view only applied to the "urban, middle-and upper-caste, middle-and upper-class Hindu and Muslim women," many of who practiced purdah strictly. See Lal, "The Politics of Gender and Medicine in Colonial India," 38–41.
5. Lal, "The Politics of Gender and Medicine in Colonial India," 57.
6. In the present chapter, I identify the literature on maternity health in colonial India of which Burma was a constitutional part until 1937. For literature on other colonies, see, for example, Hilary Marland, "Midwives, Missions and Reform: Colonizing Dutch Childbirth Services at Home and Abroad ca. 1900," in *Medicine and Colonial Identity*, edited by Mary P.Sutpan and Bridie Andersons (London: Routledge, 2003), 61–78.
7. Marchioness of Dufferin and Ava, *Our Viceregal Life in India: Selection from My Journal 1884–1888* (New York: Charles Scribner's Sons, 1891), 197.
8. *Notes and Statistics of the Hospitals and Dispensaries in Burma, for the Year 1900* (Rangoon: Office of the Superintendent, Government Printing, Burma, 1901), 2.
9. Judith L. Richell, *Disease and Demography in Colonial Burma* (Singapore: National University of Singapore Press, 2006), 85–106.
10. Lal, "Countess of Dufferin's Fund," 49.
11. Thomas Franklin Pedley, "Midwifery among the Burmese," *Transactions of the Obstetrical Society of London* 39 (1887): 8.
12. Maria Collins Douglass, "The Medical Practice and Obstetrics of the Burmese and Karens." Collection: Record of W/MCP Medical Students 1850–1981(ACC-072), Item Number: a072_1882 Douglass (Archives & Special Collections, Drexel University College of Medicine, 1882), 19–21.
13. Pedley, "Midwifery among the Burmese," 9, 10, 12.
14. Douglass, "The Medical Practice and Obstetrics of the Burmese and Karens," 25–26.
15. Pedley, "Midwifery among the Burmese," 10.
16. Douglass, "The Medical Practice and Obstetrics of the Burmese and Karens," 23.
17. Pedley, "Midwifery among the Burmese," 11.
18. Douglass, "The Medical Practice and Obstetrics of the Burmese and Karens," 24.
19. Pedley, "Midwifery among the Burmese," 11.
20. Pedley, "Midwifery among the Burmese," 11.

21. Douglass, "The Medical Practice and Obstetrics of the Burmese and Karens," 25.
22. Douglass, "The Medical Practice and Obstetrics of the Burmese and Karens," 24.
23. Pedley, "Midwifery among the Burmese," 7–8.
24. Pedley, "Midwifery among the Burmese," 7–8.
25. Atsuko Naono, "Inoculators, the Indigenous Obstacle to Vaccination in Colonial Burma," *Journal of Burma Studies* 14 (2010): 91–114.
26. Douglass, "The Medical Practice and Obstetrics of the Burmese and Karens," 21–22.
27. Pedley, "Midwifery among the Burmese," 8, 13. Dr. Pedley also states that tetanus to be the cause of mother's deaths labor is unknown in "parturient European women" and he is informed that tetanus cases are also rare in "parturient women in India" (13, 15).
28. Pedley, "Midwifery among the Burmese," 7.
29. Keith Norman MacDonald, *The Practice of Medicine among the Burmese, Translated from Original Manuscripts with an Historical Sketch of the Progress of Medicine, from the Earliest Times* (Edinburgh: MacLachlan and Stewart, 1879), 55.
30. Rosemary Fitzgerald, "'Clinical Christianity': The Emergence of Medical Work as a Missionary Strategy in Colonial India, 1800–1914," *Health, Medicine, and Empire: Perspectives on Colonial India*, edited by Biswamoy Pati and Mark Harrison (New Delhi: Orient Longman, 2001), 97–102; Maung Shwe Wa, Genevieve Sowards, and Erville Sowards, *Burma Baptist Chronicle* (Rangoon: University Press, 1963), 145.
31. Shwe Wa, Sowards, and Sowards, *Burma Baptist Chronicle*, 240.
32. Mrs. Henry G. Safford, *The Golden Jubilee* (New York: Woman's American Baptist Mission Society, 1914), 58. It is reported that, in the first year, Mitchell taught this class to "English-speaking women." Though it did not clarify the ethnicity of these women, it is possible that these included some of the Christianized indigenous women who had already received English education.
33. Safford, *The Golden Jubilee*, 58.
34. Safford, *The Golden Jubilee*, 58; *Our Medical Work in the Orient* (New York: The General Board of Promotion of the Northern Baptist Convention for the Women's American Baptist Foreign Mission Society, 1921), 29–30.
35. Randolph L. Howard, ed. *Baptists in Burma* (Philadelphia: The Judson Press, 1931), 100.
36. Edith V. Blackwell, "Nursing in Burma," *American Journal of Nursing* 38, no. 10 (1938): 1080.
37. Blackwell, "Nursing in Burmah," *British Medical Journal* (March 17, 1888): 604.
38. *Helping Hand* 27–28 (1898), 117; Safford, *The Golden Jubilee*, pp. 59–60; Shwe Wa, Sowards, and Sowards, *Burma Baptist Chronicle*, 245.
39. Blackwell, "Nursing in Burmah," 604.
40. *Triennial Report on Hospitals and Dispensaries in Burma, for the Years 1902 to 1904* (Rangoon: Office of the Superintendent, Government Printing, Burma, 1905), 7.
41. *The Nursing Record & Hospital World* (7 May 1898), 384.
42. *The Nursing Record & Hospital World* (2 December 1899), 447.
43. *The Nursing Record & Hospital World* (20 January 1900), 59.
44. A letter from (Sd.) George Hamilton to Sir Hugh Barnes, Lieutenant Governor of Burma on 9 July 1903. Mss Eur F123/72.
45. A letter from (Sd.) George Hamilton to Sir Hugh Barnes, Lieutenant Governor of Burma on 2 September 1903. Mss Eur F123/72.
46. Sometimes her first name is wrongly given as Mary. However, the relative of May Fowler-Thompson confirmed her first name as May. I thank Rick Cooper, her descendant, for clarifying this.
47. *Baptist Missionary Magazine* 78, no. 5 (May 1898): 172; A. M. Bacon, *Twenty Years' History of the Women's Baptist Foreign Missionary Society of the West* (n.p.: Women's Baptist Foreign Missionary Society of the West, 1891), 27.
48. Safford, *The Golden Jubilee*, 100.
49. Blackwell, "Nursing in Burmah," 604.
50. "Medical News," *British Medical Journal* (May 28, 1892), 1172.
51. *Notes and Statistics on the Hospitals and Dispensaries in Burma, for the Year 1900*, 2.

52. *Notes and Statistics on the Hospitals and Dispensaries in Burma, for the Year 1902*, 2.
53. *Notes and Statistics on the Hospitals and Dispensaries in Burma, for the Year 1906*, 16.
54. "Resolution on the Triennial Report on the Hospitals and Dispensaries of Burma for the Year 1905 to 1907," *Triennial Report on the Hospitals and Dispensaries of Burma for the Year 1905 to 1907*.
55. *Triennial Report on the Hospitals and Dispensaries of Burma, for the Year 1905 to 1907*, 10.
56. *Triennial Report on the Hospitals and Dispensaries of Burma, for the Year 1908 to 1910*, 13.
57. Lal, "The Politics of Gender and Medicine in Colonial India," 45.
58. *Report on the Working of the Government Medical School, Rangoon, for the Year 1917–1918* (Rangoon: Office of the Superintendent, Government Printing, Burma, 1918), 3. According to the same report for 1907 to 1921, the expenditure for the travel allowance to the students increased from 456–4–6 rupees in 1907 to 7504–10–0 rupees in 1920.
59. *Notes and Statistics on Hospitals and Dispensaries in Burma, for the Year 1908*, 3; *Notes and Statistics on Hospitals and Dispensaries in Burma, for the Year 1909*, 2.
60. "Baby Show at Sagaing," *The Rangoon Gazette*, 10 January 1916, 45.
61. Richell, *Disease and Demography in Colonial Burma*, 123. However, one of the newspapers reported that Captain Rost from the IMS led the organization of the Society for the Prevention of Infantile Mortality in Burma in 1906 by convincing leading Burmese in Rangoon to join. "The Burma Baby Show at Rangoon," *Eastern Daily Mail and Straits Morning Advertiser*, 25 June 1907, 1–4.
62. See Atsuko Naono for the health educational activities of the Burma Branch of the Red Cross. Naono, "Burmese Health Officers in the Transformation of Public Health in Colonial Burma in the 1920s and 1930s," in *Public Health in the British Empire: Intermediaries, Subordinates, and Public Health Practice, 1850–1960*, edited by Ryan Johnson and Amna Khalid (New York: Routledge, forthcoming).
63. Mr. H. F. Searle, Settlement Officer, no. III Party. *Burma Gazetteer Mandalay District Volume A* (Rangoon: Superintendent, Government Printing and Stationery, 1928), 223–24.
64. *Abstract of the Proceedings of the Council of the Lieutenant-Governor of Burma, Assembled for the Purpose of Making Laws and Regulations under the Provisions of the Government of India Act*. 5 April 1922, 1015–18.
65. For example, Richell explains, in Maymyo, that it took ten more years for this act to be applied when the *wan zwe* were prohibited to practice. See Richell, *Disease and Demography in Colonial Burma*, 125.
66. For example, Richell analyzed that the trained midwives attended only 3.86 percent of mothers in the countryside in 1939. See Richell, *Disease and Demography in Colonial Burma*, 124.
67. Nellie G. Prescott, *The Baptist Family in Foreign Mission Fields* (New York: Department of Missionary Education, Board of Education, the Northern Baptist Convention, 1926): 48–49.
68. Ma Saw Sa, *Midwifery* (Rangoon: Burma Union, 1921).
69. *Our Medical Work in the Orient* (New York: The General Board of Promotion of the Northern Baptist Convention for the Women's American Baptist Foreign Mission Society, 1921), 33; Prescott, *The Baptist Family in Foreign Mission Fields*, 63.

Chapter Eight

Unani Medical Culture

Memory, Representation, and the Literate Critical Anticolonial Public Sphere

Neshat Quaiser

In a resistance to Western medical epistemological absolutism and the representation of the self-image of Unani medicine, during the colonial period, memory and representation were key defining categories that enabled Unani medicine to create a specific niche for itself within the *critical anticolonial* public sphere,[1] which was dominated by elite and literate practitioners and other votaries of Unani. The debate, with memory as one of the key elements, exceeded simple medical and health considerations producing combative modes of representation related to medicine and health practices, as also the ways in which these were inextricably linked with the larger sociocultural and economic interests, and the colonial culture of domination. Memory, however, was not fabricated or invented in the strict sense of the term,[2] but was characterized by the employment and assertion of *high facts* against the colonially driven fabrication of the Unani past. In other words, Unani traditions of the then recent origin were not given an entirely invented continuity with a historic past. With elite and other literate classes dominating the scene, memory was employed to strategically popularize the high facts as pan Indian Muslim remembrance to face the colonial and to project a united Unani whole. Memory and representation, thus, were strategies where the part intended to implicate the whole. However, despite limitations, the literate Unani resistance to Western medical absolutism constituted a significant visible presence in the encounter and exchange between the two systems of medicine.

The question of encounter between indigenous and Western medicine during the colonial period has often been questioned by various scholars. Langford[3], following Taussig,[4] has argued that it was not encounter but a kind of mimesis. Recently, Mukharji[5] has forcefully questioned the idea of encounter where colonial state patronized Western medicine and denigrated indigenous medicine in India and that the relationship between the two medical practices was marked by encounter. However, despite a certain "localization and 'Unani-ization' of Western medicine,"[6] opposition to the ideological hegemony of Western medicine remained a dominant trend on the part of Unani even on disciplinary grounds. It is important to note that the relationship between the two knowledge systems during the colonial period was characterized by both encounter and exchange—Unani did not hesitate to learn from Western medicine, and the colonial state did not hesitate, or was forced, to employ Unani to meet the health needs.

This chapter examines the ways in which Western medicine and Unani were represented and self-represented within the arena of professional and non-professional literate Unani medical culture[7] that significantly molded the nature of encounters between the two systems. More importantly, the organizing principles of self-defense and Unani's critical representations of Western medicine emanated from the *retentionist* internal logic of its own existence that developed a critical ethico-cultural logic of resistance. Thus, Unani medical culture was prominently marked by an *informed* conscience based on ethical values, associated traditionally with the profession of tibb, which formed the key structuring principle to critique the colonially propelled, market-oriented logic of Western medicine.[8] The troubled encounter between the two medical systems further concretized the critical anticolonial public sphere.

Unani medical culture in colonial India was essentially *dispersed* and inclusive in nature, and was a component of *Medical Public Sphere.*[9] This culture was characterized by a sense of injustice done to Unani by Western medical absolutism through colonial machinations; a conscience-based ethical value system for the medical profession; a plea for human knowledge as shared heritage; a critique of the capitalist market logic of Western medicine; endeavors to validate the present through the strategies of memory, reminder, and representation, public debate on science, health, body, rationality, modernism, Eurocentrism, Western education, and economic exploitation; upholding Unani's medico-cultural identity; and defiance as the dominant mood in the face of colonial might but also readiness to learn from others.

UNANI MEDICINE AND INDIAN CONNECTIONS

Unani medicine refers to the Greco-Arab system of medicine as it developed in the Indian subcontinent since the twelfth century AD. Prior to its introduction in the Indian subcontinent, it also benefited from the traditional knowledge systems in Egypt, Syria, Iraq, China, and other Middle East and Far East societies. Just before the advent of Western medicine, Unani medicine was immensely popular, widely practiced, and used over the vast territory of the Indian subcontinent[10] and continued to be so even after the introduction of Western medicine under colonial patronage.[11] Hippocrates, the Greek philosopher-physician, was the founder of the Unani system of medicine and is believed to have freed medicine from the realm of superstition and magic to give it the status of science. The theoretical framework of Unani is based on the teachings of Hippocrates. Galen (AD 131–210), following Hippocrates, is known to have consolidated its foundation on which Arab physicians like Abu Bakr Muhammad bin Zakariyya ar-Razi (Rhazes) (AD 850–925) and Abu 'Ali Husain bin Abdullah bin Sina, popularly known as Ibn Sina (Avicenna, AD 980–1036) built a magnificent and durable structure.

The earliest of the Arab medical scholars was Ali b. Rabban, who, in AD 850, in his book, *Firdausul-Hikmat* (*Paradise of Wisdom*), summarized the whole system of Greek medicine as well as the Indian system of medicine on the basis of four important Indian medical works—by Caraka, Susruta, Nidana, and Astangahrdaya. Following him, his student, Abu Bakr Muhammad bin Zakariyya ar-Razi (Rhazes), studied the two systems, and as in charge of several local hospitals, introduced the system of records of each case with focus on the practical training of students. Bahwa bin Khwas Khan's *Ma'dan al-Shifa-e Sikandar Shahi* written in the period of Sikander Lodhi (1489–1517), is an important text depicting the inclusive nature of Unani. However, Ibn Sina (Avicenna) continues to be one of the most important early scholars of medicine. His Qanun (Canon Medicinae) was accepted as the most authoritative medical work in Europe from the twelfth to seventeenth centuries, as well as in India to present day. Improved and systematized by Arab scholars, Unani medicine was introduced in India in the twelfth century AD with Ziauddin Ahmad Aburrafe Hiravi from Herat as the first physician, renowned for his medical skills, appointed under Sultan Khusrau Malik (1160–1186) of Lahore.[12] It flourished throughout the Indian subcontinent for eight hundred years, beginning from the Sultanate Period (1206–1413), and later was patronized by Muslim rulers and nobles, as is evident from the large number of hospitals they built for the people. Practitioners of Ayurveda and Unani continued to practice in the hospitals founded by the Mughal rulers.[13]

After the fall of the Mughal empire, the Unani system came under the patronage of Nawabs and nobles of princely states and elites, and continued to enjoy popularity among the masses. Alongside the established city-based families of hakims (practitioners of Unani medicine), there were many small town families and individual hakims who were traditionally associated with the practice of Unani in almost every part of the country; these families and individuals significantly contributed to the promotion of this system in the face of the onslaught launched by Western medicine, as is evident from the various accounts on the history and practice of Unani in the subcontinent. These families owned several *Matabs* (clinics), imparting education to enthusiastic students who successfully practiced medicine after completing their training from Matabs. The trained hakims were not always from an elite background; many of them belonged to middle and lower middle class families.

MEMORY, REPRESENTATION, THE PAST, AND THE QUESTION OF RECOVERY

Memory assumed a strategic site for Unani medicine in its struggle against Western medicine. Memory in the given context was crucially rooted in an idea of recovery—recovery of what was lost in a real or perceived unnatural way. The idea of recovery in the case of Unani during the colonial period was both secular and Muslim/Islamic. It was secular in terms of the material base of disease and health that remained a structuring principle for Unani. It was also secular in terms of its consumers and practitioners with no religious or caste basis, in terms of accessibility to all sections of the population, and in terms of patrons including Muslim and Hindu rulers, nobles, princely states, and other affluent sections. It was Muslim/Islamic for the Muslim elite and skilled practitioners of Unani who were most visible, due to its Greco-Arab past and the influence of Islamic precepts in the practice of Unani. Viewed thus, recovery was a critical site for the "Muslim" political struggle against colonialism engaging Unani as part of this struggle.

With the advent of colonialism and Western medicine, the recovery of the lost status and prestige, perceived thus, became the prime concern for the advocates of Unani. Memory, the past, and recovery of the forgotten past, thus, emerged as critical sites for Unani in a struggle with recovery directed toward self-criticality and the spirit of learning.

In contemporary social science scholarship, the question of interpretation and reinterpretation of facts, the past, and history have come to occupy a defining place. The shifting meanings of facts and history are mediated by the ways in which a host of social forces view these aspects in accordance with how they affect them in the present time. Arguments and counterarguments have been marshalled both in favor of the sanctity of historical facts and privileging actors' view of facts in the given contexts of time and space. The past constructed through the present and the present constructed through the past have emerged as constituting a binary opposition. In the midst of this controversy, one thing is clear: the role played by extra-fact considerations in the constitution of perceptions and identities, both individual and collective, in everyday life has often, if not always, created a situation of political arbitrariness in the conceptions of both past and facts. However, the radical strategy of construction of the present through the past in the case of Unani did not always produce a binary opposition between past and present but a critical synthesis.

Memory, representation, and public sphere together constituted a complex whole in the context of Western-Unani encounter in colonial India. Memory, history, and the past (among others) were necessary weapons to counter the colonial projects to hegemonize the public spheres to sustain the relations of domination. In the context of Unani-Western medicine, Unani practitioners projected the past as living present. Memory was not simply to authenticate the past but as something that validated the present as systems of *parallel* practice and meaning.[14] The terrain of memory emerged as a crucial defining element in the constitution of Unani's representation of the self and Western medicine, and in the constitution of a Unani medical entity. In the resistance to hegemony of Western medical absolutism, the present was mediated by the past with a view of the future. Memory became one of the crucial mechanisms for reclaiming the desired past and collective self for a desired present and future. There occurred a kind of institutionalization of memory and it emerged as conceptually and operationally instrumental. In this whole process of the play of memory and the past in the public spheres, the modes of representations became crucial political and cultural acts for both domination and resistance, as was evident in the encounter between Unani and Western medicine.[15] This act of critiquing heralded a reverse process of representation of Western medicine by Unani.

A general operational mechanism of representation involving the colonized and the colonizer evolved a certain pattern of image-making even in the encounter of Unani and Western medicine. The mechanism had two sets of separate but connected modes of representation: first, colonial representation of self-image and the colonial representation of the colonized; and second, representation of the self-image and of the colonizer by the colonized, all of which took place through and against each other.

The colonial state and its ideological apparatuses made constant efforts to occupy nearly all the available public spheres that had the potential of being anticolonial. But the technologies of domination never remained completely uncontested, paving the way for the emergence and strengthening of a critical anticolonial public sphere. The colonial power projected not only its own medical knowledge as modern, authentic, scientific, and superior but also appropriated the right to interpret and represent the medical knowledge of the colonized people. Such colonial representations produced both conformity and contestation. Economic and political factors underlying such assertions enable us to critique the views that "colonialism itself was a cultural project" and empire was all about cultural interactions.[16] For interaction was hardly "dialogic" at an institutional level; colonial domination, instead, produced largely asymmetrical relations of power between the colonized and the colonizer at all levels of the Unani-Western medicine encounter.

An important feature of the resultant strategies of representation was that instead of getting "constructed" in the image of the West, Unani attempted to construct Europe and Western medicine in its own image. Edward Said had once argued that imperialism constructed the colonial world in its own image. The Saidian understanding of the role of imperialism with its heavy accent on the "radiation" factor, where the colonial subjects appear almost as a passive mass, has come in for sharp criticism.[17] However, it is not simply the question of passivity but the reverse process of construction and representation that assumed greater significance in this regard.

UNANI AND THE SCIENCE QUESTION IN COLONIAL INDIA

Studies on social history of medicine of colonial India have addressed the question of medicine in colonial India and colonial medicine from the perspective of colonial requirements of expansion using medicine as a means of domination. Similarly, the question of science in colonial India and of colonial science has attracted the attention of scholars such as George Basalla, Donald Fleming, Daniel Headrick, Roy MacLeod, Deepak Kumar, and Mark Harrison,[18] among others, in a significant way. But the science in the domain of medicine and the debate around it in colonial India have yet to receive adequate response. However, debates around the question of science in the context of encounters between Indian and Western systems of medicine and its practice constitute an area of inquiry that needs attention.[19]

Western science in colonial India has largely been viewed as colonial science.[20] Harrison, however, argues that scientific work in the British colonies has been presented as "derivative, instrumentalist, and exploitative, with colonial scientists seen as mere fact gatherers." He also argues that "science came to be seen in the colonies increasingly as an instrument of imperial control rather than the key to development," claiming that recent research reveals a much richer tapestry, and questions the basic assumptions that historians have made about science in the colonies.[21] But science and medicine were largely intertwined with colonial projects of profit, of siphoning off resources and colonial control, thus projecting the science which the West had exclusively produced. Colonial power did not project science as a part of cumulative knowledge that humans acquired over a long period of time in their practical interaction with nature. Unani, for example, did not form a declared part of Western science.[22] Such an approach ruled out the possibility of understanding science and medicine through the prism of shared spaces of knowledge despite Unani's approach to benefit from recent research in Western medicine.

The question of science in colonial India was much more visible in the domain of medicine. The culture of medical science and practices in India outside the gambit of the colonial project of medicine was plural in nature. Diversity of medical knowledge and practices was influenced by cultural practices in addition to expert medical knowledge including the Unani system. It was not only plural but also significantly *dispersed* as opposed to the concentration of medical knowledge at the elite expert level. The insistence on approved and licensed standardization of medical knowledge by the colonial administration raised questions of rationality/irrationality, body, science, progress, development, East, West, and other colonially-constructed binary oppositions, responses, and counter-responses by advocates of Unani and Western medicine, and were debated at profesisonal and popular levels.

The culture of medical science existed as an integral part of Unani and was not prompted by Western medicine, as has generally been argued.[23] Scientific activities, including thinking and writing in all forms in the nineteenth and twentieth centuries, became more intense with added colonial trappings to make a point that science in medicine already existed and also to come to terms with changing times as a natural corollary. The argument of the dominant responses[24] to and critique of Western medicine was that the revitalization of Unani was not caused by the Western ideology of modernism but by its own internal logic of *renewal*. Thus, continued efforts were made at retaining the fundamental principles of Unani not only as medical knowledge and culture, but also for the economic interests of its practitioners and patrons. Through various representational strategies, it was vehemently contested that Unani was unscientific and irrational; to this effect, renewal of the Unani system included restoration of and learning from new "scientific" methods without altering its fundamentals. Thus, the reform endeavor was considered essentially to be informed renewal.[25] The debate outlined the process of coming to terms with one's own self in a colonially structured unexpected situation.

UNANI MEDICAL CULTURE AND THE LITERATE CRITICAL ANTICOLONIAL PUBLIC SPHERE

The debate on the public sphere in recent times has largely been centered on Habermas's pioneering work on the subject. His concept of public sphere was rooted in the historical experiences of Western bourgeois society and absolutist state, based on the conceptual distinction between state and civil society where the existence of a political community and its political autonomy from the state was a primary concern.[26] Historical contexts of public spheres in colonies, however, were different from that of Western bourgeois society. In India, there existed multiple public spheres encompassing almost all the aspects of social life representing conflicting ideological orientations where the political was one significant aspect. These were marked by various traditional, formal and informal, and critical and conformist modes of communication outside the state, with internal divisions.

With the advent of colonial encounters and rule, Western dimensions of ideas relating to individuals as citizens, science and rationality, individualism, freedom, modernism, state and society, and print culture also began to manifest in public spheres in the Indian subcontinent, which is evident from the Unani medical culture as well. With the widespread machinations of colonial rule, public sphere in India acquired new dimensions with colonial and anticolonial trappings. The literate critical anticolonial public sphere (within critical anticolonial public sphere) was accommodative on secular and democratic lines. It was literate because of its reliance on a canonized tradition and was largely composed of *khandani* hakims that looked down upon non-*khandani* who were not formally trained hakims. Nevertheless, it was close to the nationalist public sphere.[27] The critical anticolonial public sphere was, thus, directed toward subversion of colonial machinations of control alongside class- and caste-based relations of domination. The nationalist public sphere, fraught with contradictions, was influenced by colonial constructs of modernism, scientific, and democratic civilization, and also by the local feudal and class relations. Such trends led to *locational determinism*, where unchangeable conformity to collective representations becomes inevitable.[28] However, the organizing principles of the Unani literate critical anticolonial public sphere were not wholly structured through and against Western modernism. For instance, Unani's intense opposition to Western medical absolutism and critique of colonial representations of the medical knowledge of the colonized occupied a prominent place within this public sphere as it emanated from its internal logic of renewal. Moreover, the place of Unani in this sphere was natural as the regular nationalist public sphere of powerful forces such as the Congress and Gandhi, paid no heed to issues concerning indigenous medicine despite the mounting pressure from Western medicine that had emerged as a tool of colonial domination.

The domain of medicine was, perhaps, the most compelling site for the articulation of sentiments against the claims of superiority of Western knowledge. Western medicine saw Unani medicine as irrational and unscientific, thus heightening the pressure on Unani to reform accordingly. Theoretically, colonial politics of comparison was at work behind such assumptions. This increased hostility between the two systems and led to a commotion within Unani medical culture at all levels—the elite, non-elite practitioners, Unani clientele, and the educated votaries of Unani. In this respect, learning from others was justified through a representation of the spirit of knowledge-seeking based on Islamic precepts.[29] As Altaf Husayn Hālī, a famous Urdu poet and reformer, asserted:

Ki Hikmat Ko Aik Ġumšudah L'l Samjho
Jahan Pāo Apnā Ause Māl Samjho

(Knowledge be considered the lost ruby.
Wherever you find it take it as your own property.)[30]

Such a representation of knowledge, in fact, in a way also contested the strict "internalist"[31] view of science and knowledge. Unani's debate with Western medicine was intrinsically linked with the overall chaotic sociopolitical situation that heightened after the second half of the nineteenth century. Increasing pressure within Unani medical culture to adopt western standards of education, medicine, literature, the arts, and such, was quite palpable.[32] Sir Syed Ahmad Khan was severely criticized for his advocacy of English education and Western medicine. Akbar Allahabadi, a very well-known Urdu writer, poet, public figure, and a contemporary of Sir Syed, captured the mood prevailing against Sir Syed, English education, and Western medicine in the following couplets:

'ql Sapurd-e-Māstar, Māl Sapurd-e-Ānjanāb
Jān Sapurd-e-Dāctar, Ruh Sapurd-e-Darwin
Jān Šāyad Farištay Chor Bhī Dīn
Dāctar Fīs Ko Nah Chorīngī
Dāctar Sāhab Sī Milnā Āp Ka ačha Nahīn
Baythī Ghar Mīn Mujhī Bīmār Rāhnī Dījiye.

(Intellect is surrendered to master [teacher] and
wealth to Your Honour.
Life is surrendered to doctor and soul to Darwin.
Angels may grant life,
But doctors will never agree to forego their fees.

It is not good for me to meet doctor sāhab.
It is better that I sit back at home and remain sick.)[33]

A reading of the above couplets reveals certain shifts within the social life with the advent of entrenched colonialism. To this effect, Akbar Allahabadi argued that independent thinking was being surrendered to the modern English education and medicine[34] with indigenous material resources and wealth being siphoned off to Britain. Besides, Western medicine and its practitioners were guided by the colonial capitalist market logic, which was in direct conflict with the ethical values traditionally associated with the profession of *tibb*.[35] Similarly, debates on anticolonial sentiments coupled with anticolonial struggles were also reflected in the Unani medical culture, best seen in the founding of the All India Vaidik and Unani Tibbī Conference (AIVUTC) in 1906, with claims to jointly represent Unani and Ayurveda[36] against the challenges posed by Western medicine. In the fifth meeting of the conference held at Patna, a poet hailed the unity efforts as follows:

Tibb Ke Āīne Men Yun Jalwa-e-Vaidik Hay 'ayān
Jays e Shīshe Men Parī Ko Leta Haī Koī Utar
Phūl Chun Kar Tibb Se Jo Gundhe Gaye The
Aaj Wo Shāyad āyurved Ke Gale Men Hayn Hār

(The image of āyurvayd is so prominent in the
mirror of Unani Tibb as though one has captivated a
fairy. The garland woven with the flowers of Tibb is
put round the neck of āyurvayd.)[37]

Despite efforts at unity hailed in the above couplets, Unani medical culture faced professional rivalry not only from Western medicine but also with its counterpart, Ayurveda. This was not just professional rivalry; it also betrayed historical-political power relations and its wider acceptability in the late nineteenth century as well as the simmering communalization under colonial rule. Moreover, a play of memory and representation is palpable and the antiquity of Unani and its global significance remembered and reminded to establish *tibb*'s independent identity. Nevertheless, due to its location within the critical anticolonial public sphere, practitioners of Unani and Ayurved joined in their anticolonial struggle. For example, in the unity efforts between Unani and Ayurveda, it was suggested:

Aik Aur Aik Milne Se Hue Gyarah Hayn
Tibb Ho Vaidic Ki Madad-gār Pau-barah Hain

(One plus one can make eleven.
If tibb renders aid to Vaidic, we will come off
successful.)[38]

Similarly, Western medicine was reminded and advised:

> *Tum Jo Munkir Hue Arbon Kī Kamai Se Ho*
> *Hai Juda Dāktary Kahte Dhitaī Se Ho*
> *Kawnsī Hūbi Hay Tujh Men Jo Tibābat Men Nahīn*
> *Fāidah Kuč̌h Bhi Merī Jān Raqābat Men Nahīn*
>
> (You deny but whatever you are, it is due to the achievements of Arabs. With audacity and effrontery you declare daktary is separate. What are the virtues that you have, which Unani medical art does not have? There is no use for rivalry, my dear.)[39]

Implicit in both couplets is the message of treating human knowledge as commonly shared heritage. Defiance, thus, seemed to be the dominant mood. History and memory as constant defining conceptual tools were deployed as a necessary reminder. For instance:

> *Tibb Thī Majbūr Faqat Be-sar-o-sāmāni Men*
> *Varna Thī Dāktary Āpki Kis Pānī Men*
> *Band Šīše Men Vilāyat Se Pari Āī*
> *Lāl Pīlī Huī, Ġusse Men Bharī Āī*
> *Chaman-e-Tibb Se Guldastah Ura Kar Lāī*
> *Naī Tarkīb Se Bandish Sajā Kar Lāī*
>
> (Tibb was constrained owing to lack of means, otherwise what was the worth of Western medicine. In a closed bottle a fairy has come full of anger from foreign lands. The bouquet [Western medicine] stolen from the garden of [Unani] Tibb has been rearranged in a new fashion.)[40]

The above couplets critique the colonial character of Western medicine for being like a "bouquet stolen from the garden of *tibb* rearranged in a new fashion." There is also a critique of the market-oriented capitalist art of packaging goods to attract customers and opposition to it.

Unani medical culture and the general public sphere in colonial India were replete with several deeper questions with far-reaching implications for modernity, the notion of time, and for Western medicine and Unani. For instance, Hakim Firuz al-Dīn provided an extremely significant representation of why people were attracted to Western medicine instead of Unani. He went into the domain of public social life and the ways in which it was affected by "modern education" and the colonial system. He said:

> In India, modern education is fast spreading. And the requirements of life of Indians have expanded so much that they get little rest, peace and satisfaction. Moreover, in their nature, a kind of hastiness has come into existence, the inevitable result of which is that their mental faculties cannot function fully. They always desire that whatever problems they are faced with should come to an end immediately with either good or bad results. If there is any obstacle in the fixed routine of their lives that should be removed fast. This is the reason that whenever they fall sick they run towards the direction from where they can recover fast without any thinking about what will be the final result of it.[41]

Hakim Firuz al-Dīn's explanation is extremely instructive. It reveals the tectonic shift in Indian social life emphasizing that the notion of time underwent a fundamental change with the capitalist-colonial notion permeating into the Indian public sphere and hence routinizing everyday life; this was to alter the notion of work paving the way for utilitarian rationality. Besides, we find that a critique of European modernity as "the modern" is also inherent in the argument. Together, they created a situation where the "mental faculties" of people "could not function fully," and they ran "toward the direction from where they could recover fast" during sickness.

The colonial-capitalist notion of time and work emerged from a system of individual responsibility for "getting the work done"; in India, this notion produced *feudocracy* and *feudocratic* structures. Capitalist bureaucracy in the Western contexts, as Weber explained, was based on rational legal authority. In India, colonial power introduced bureaucracy modeled after the Western pattern and an advanced industrial network, although in the absence of a capitalist mode of production, the capitalist work ethics and notion of time could not be fully inculcated. This produced *feudocracy* and *feudocratic* structures, characterized by Western legality of target-oriented work ethics as well as the feudal notion of work ethics of caste-class divisions and hierarchical patron-client relations, which formed the core of bureaucracy in colonial, as also in postcolonial India.

Charges were leveled[42] against the "inadequacies" in Unani in terms of medical training. Pressure from these charges with full support from the colonial state was very high. The impact of colonial policies was widely felt and debated publicly. Guided by the conscience-based ethical values as the structuring principle, questions of medical ethics and concern for the poor formed part of the politics of representation by advocates of Unani. Criticism against Western doctors and hospitals serving only the elite, continued unabated. Apparent lack of government support to Unani, and lack of jobs for hakims contributed to a lack of proper education in Unani medicine.[43] In addition to public figures,[44] writers, hakims, and the public actively participated in the debate. Some suggested a combination of Western medicine and Unani *tibb* to draw government support[45] while others suggested reliance on traditional knowledge and resources.

As a challenge from Western medicine as a colonial form of knowledge, the self-representation of Unani took different forms. Religious and ethical values were invoked in these public responses and representations with a critical outlook of Western medicine as also self-criticism. Deputy Nazīr Ahmed, a famous Urdu novelist in a lamenting mode of critical self-representation, complained:

> *Yah Watan Ahl-e-Watan Se Hay Nang*
> *Apne Men Lete Nahīn Ahl-e Firang*
>
> (Its own people disgrace this country.
> The foreigners do not count
> us as one of them.)[46]

Nazīr Ahmed reminded us how our *Qawm* (here, Muslim community) was great in every sphere of life, and lamented how backward we have now become, forgetting our great ancestors, and how others (colonial rulers) have made us fight against each other. He added:

> *Unke Jo Dekhe Hayn Nam ū ne Bure*
> *Pahle Se Ham Ho Gay Dūne Bure*
> *Aaysa Bhī Hotā Hay Koī Bewafā*
> *Apne Buzurgon Se Yehān Tak Hafā*
> *Dast-e-nigar Ġayron Ke Har Kār Men*
> *Kaisā Kasād Aa Gaya Bāzār Men*
>
> (Having seen their [foreigners] bad
> practices we have become still worse.
> How ungrateful we have been to our
> ancestors that they have become target of
> our anger. What a decline has come to stay
> that for everything we are dependent on
> foreigners.)[47]

Nazīr Ahmed remained critical of the British government and their political maneuvers while representing their knowledge as superior at the same time; he expressed resentment against the popular acceptance of the English language and dependence on the British. In an act of self-representation, he advocated self-reliance and community efforts to raise funds, which meant no dependence on the colonial state for the promotion and development of the Unani system.[48] He had envisaged that popular participation and willingness would bring about the desired changes when faced with opposition in the "age of peace and freedom," adding that

> in earlier times all progress depended on the support from empire and whatever caught the imagination of the Sultan and his Durbar, that things developed and became popular. But now is the age of peace and freedom. Subjects themselves can do things for the good of people that the government cannot do properly.[49]

While self-representation was rife with tensions, the power of Western medicine as a superior form of knowledge was profoundly felt at the time; it produced an increase in self-representation even in those trained in Western medicine but educated Unani. For instance, Doctor Hakim Ġulām Jīlani was concerned about bridging the gap between the two systems by introducing "scientific" elements into Unani so that its medicine and its practice could be standardized and could meet the challenges of modern times.[50] Several others shared the view. It is interesting to note that Jīlani advocated both Western medicine and Unani in his practice—playing the role of both Western doctor and hakim; he also suggested a combination of the two systems.[51]

In the politics of representation and counter representation, surgery and anatomy were at the center of debate between Western medicine and Unani from the very beginning. Under mounting pressure on the issues of lack of surgery in Unani, in his efforts to renew (as opposed to reform) and reshape medical knowledge, Hakim Ajmal Khān reacted sharply against the ignorance of Western representation in this regard.[52] Similarly, Hakim Jogī captured the sentiments on the issue of Western representation of the status of surgery in Unani by employing the strategy of memory in the following popular poetic idiom:

Ab khabardār Rahen Tibb Ko Mitāne Wāle
Jā-o-Bejā Kisī Bekas Ko Dabāne Wāle
Nāmukammal Woh Mukammal Ko Batāne Wāle
Nirī Jarrahī Pe Sau Nāz Dikhāne Wāle
Kawnsī Bāt Nikāli Thī Jigarkārī Se
Chīrnā Phārna Sīkhā Hay Yeh Zuhrāvī Se[53]

(Beware, those who seek to eliminate Unani Tibb; those who declare a complete [science] as incomplete and take pride merely on barber-surgery. They have not achieved anything from their own hard labour for they learned dissection from Zuhravi.)[54]

Similarly, colonial representation in establishing new Western medical colleges aroused sentiments about establishing colleges for both Ayurveda and Unani. A poet hakim represented the issue:

Ab Bhi Jāge Ho To Kučh Kar Dikhā Dījiyegā
Desi Tibb Ke Liye Kālij To Banā Dījiyegā
Āj Vaidik Ko Tabābat Se Milā Dījiyegā
Jān Ki Hayr Ko Ab Māl Lutā Dījiyegā

Ham Banā Dālenge Kālij Yeh Tahayyah Karlo
Tandurustī Ke Yah Sāmān Muhayyah Karlo

(Since now you are awake, do something, and
build colleges for indigenous medical sciences.
Bring Vaidic and Unani together, and for life's sake
do not hesitate to spend your wealth. For our health
we should be determined to establish colleges.)[55]

The establishment of the Tibbiya College of Delhi—a continuity of the Madras-e Tibbiya (school for Unani medicine) established in 1889, was also intricately linked with the question of the nature of science and scientific temper in colonial India. This was, perhaps, the most articulated critique of Western medicine within Unani medical culture. The College marked defiance to the medical epistemological absolutism with a key element of the logic of the colonial relations of domination. It was a significant project to claim, counterclaim, and reclaim with reference to Western and Unani medical knowledge which brought prominence to the question of recovery. Defenders of Unani refused to accept the perceived irrationality in Unani, a position that was undeniably proven and articulated by the Tibbiya College.[56] Thus, the college constituted a significant part of the critical anticolonial public sphere that challenged the colonial knowledge based on European Enlightenment of notions of modernity and progress. It defended non-European knowledge systems, defying the written and unwritten rules to fit into the ideological paradigms of the colonizers.

The science question in colonial India inspired fresh thoughts of an independent logic of existence within Unani medical culture. Despite the colonial hegemony in science, it produced significant "unintended consequences" as seen in the localization and Unani-ization of Western medicine based on the perceived historicity and heritage of Unani. Similarly, the Unani and Tibbya College and its research wing, the *Hindustaniī Dawakhana*, the *Zenana Madrasa* and the *Zenana Shifakhana*, also called *tibbi* Institutions,[57] added to these perceptions with reorganized curricula, finances, and modes of examination. The latter were based on the new contexts of colonialism, medicine, market, sciences, and the shortcomings which needed to be overcome for renewal, also indicating the limitations in the logic of modern market-oriented professional concerns.

The Unani-Western medicine debate was not confined to professionals alone. At the popular level, too, there was active participation in the ensuing discussions on medical encounters, in stories by word of mouth and through popular magazines and journals. These also became part of popular folklore memory and Unani medical culture. Besides, constant representations of patients as getting back to Unani after disappointments with *Daktary* formed an integral part of popular Unani medical culture. From these encounters emerged specific modes of counter representation of the self and the other that were used to defy Western medicine, facilitated by the new print culture.

In an Urdu medical journal, one hakim, Wahīd al-Haqq, a *tabīb* in the employment of Bakhtiyarpur state (Bihar), informed that on 8 July 1905, his old friend, former assistant surgeon of Madhapura, Babu Shayamapado, wrote to A'lī-Janāb Čawdhry Ajeer al-Haqq, *raīs* of Bakhtiyarpur state, District Mongyr, about Babu Braj Bansi Sahai's (Sub Divisional Officer, Madhapura, District Bhagalpur) son who was suffering from fever (*tap*) and was under his treatment. Babu Braj Bansi preferred Unani to *Dāktary* so he requested the *raīs* of Bakhtiyarpur state to send Hakim Wahīd al-Haqq, an employee of the state. Hakim Wahīd al-Haqq informed that another letter of 16 July 1905 was sent by Babu Shayamapado to the *raīs* of Bakhtiyarpur state stating that one Hakim Rashīd had come from Gaya, but requested that Hakim Wahīd al-Haqq treat him, as Western doctors were unsuccessful in treating the patient. In reply, Hakim Wahīd al-Haqq wrote,

> Hakim Rashīd wanted to give *Mus'hil* but in the presence of two *Dāktar* who were treating the patient, who would listen to Hakim Rashīd? I agreed with Hakim Rashīd and insisted on giving *mus'hil*. My opinion was liked. The boy was cured. The purpose of telling this story is that hakims should pay serious attention to the development of Unani *tibb* and nobles and those who held the reins of country and nations should pay full attention to this useful system of medical treatment. This system was noble and easily accessible and should be saved from being eliminated.[58]

In one of the Urdu Indian newspapers, a reader—one *Noon* (the Urdu alphabet indicating the first letter of his name)—wrote,

> It was an established fact that Unani *tibb* was the best of all sciences, and its usefulness was proved. It worked slowly and even if hakims committed a mistake it could be corrected. No matter how poor the patient was, medicine was administered till the end and he was not killed by administering acid. No matter how much temptation was given to the hakim, no matter how much unpleasantness was there (between the hakim and patient), but the method of treatment was such that he in no case could administer any deadly medicine to anybody.

The letter further stated,

> It was not that Unani practitioners did not commit mistakes; neither *Dāktary* nor Unani was free from mistakes . . . but Unani cured with mild medicines, their mistakes were corrected but *Dāktar*'s medicines were instantly effective and the patient became incurable even if a slight wind of mistake touched him. *Dāktary* medicines were also given on guess and because they were quick in

> effect, their victims couldn't even ask for water. The words "slow" and "quick" in the above statement clearly refer to the western and Indian pace of doing linked with the notion of time.

On the question of hakims acquiring expertise, he retorted,

> On what assurance they could complete their proper education? There was no job for them in the government. Leaders of *qawm* did not bother about them. Rich and noble did not bother about them. How would they complete their proper education? If at least in big cities, a few hakims were employed then one would see to what extent this science could develop. It would not only be wrong but absolutely wrong to apply the experiences of Paris and London: when the temperament and climate of India were different from those countries, then how could we succeed in these experiments? That was why in India the reforms those doctors kept making through their efforts and their attempts to change climate were always unsuccessful, and different types of epidemic had destroyed India.

He added,

> When a man could not get even a simple diet how could he succeed in the development of his science? Just see how doctors had been provided with all facilities for development of their science. It was a pity that India was seeing a great science in the deathbed and could not do anything.[59]

The letter is a trenchant critique of profit making as the central motive for the practitioners of Western medicine and clearly points out that conscience-based medical ethics is argued for and juxtaposed Unani medical practice to Western medical profession, which was regarded as a profit-making venture even at the cost of patients' peril. It was believed that the government did not provide adequate opportunities for Unani to prosper as a viable knowledge system. And claims for refuting that doctors can treat all diseases, that their diagnosis is complete, and that they cannot make mistakes are revealed in the following narrative:

> A man called Hudson had drowned in the river Thames in a boat tragedy. Dāktars, after examining declared him dead but two non-medical persons did not agree with them and after their efforts for about two hours Hudson was found alive. If one depended only on Dāktary then Hudson would have lost his life.[60]

These stories within Unani medical culture seriously questioned the absolutism of western medicine and constituted a prominent anticolonial signature.

In conclusion, Western medicine emerged as a crucial means for understanding colonial representations of the colonized, the colonizer, and of the colonial modes of domination. In this regard, while colonial constructions of medicine and health were imposed on India and her people, the politics of representation for Western medicine was made well nigh intricate and challenging. Resistance to Western medicine by practitioners, consumers, the general public, and leaders occupied a significant place within the Unani medical culture located within the critical anticolonial public sphere. History, the past, memory, and representation as strategies of resistance were deployed to counter and construct Western medicine. Reconstructing the past and memory as organizing principles of the debate engendered systems of parallel practice and meaning.[61] The retentionist internal logic of renewal of Unani had a lot to do with the ways in which Europe and Western medicine were represented and contested. Viewed thus, the anticolonial ideology of medicine utilized by Unani was marked by a critical ethico-cultural logic of resistance which, in turn, was guided by informed, conscience-based ethical values of Unani; the latter constituted one of the key structuring principles to critique the colonially constructed, profit-oriented market logic of Western medicine.

ACKNOWLEDGMENT

An earlier draft of this chapter was presented at the IFRI Conference (Tehran, February 2008). This chapter draws partially from Quaiser (2000). Santanu Sengupta proofread and checked the footnotes for the earlier draft-his occasional presence was reassuring. Thanks to Sayeed and Vidhi for the transcription of the diacritical marks, and to Appu Lenin for being around.

NOTES

1. Quaiser, Neshat. 2001. "Colonial Politics of Medicine and Popular *Unani* Resistance," *Indian Horizon* 47, no. 2; Quaiser, Neshat. 2011. "Science, Institution and Colonialism: Tibbiya College of Delhi, 1889–1947." In *Science in Modern India: An Institutional History, c. 1784–1947*, edited by Uma Das Gupta. Delhi: Pearson Longman.

2. Reference is to Hobsbawm, Eric J. 1983. "Introduction: Invented Tradition," in *The Invention of Tradition* by Eric J. Hobsbawm and Terence Ranger. Cambridge: Cambridge University Press.

3. Langford, Jean. 2002. *Fluent Bodies: Ayurvedic Remedies for Postcolonial Imbalance*. Durham: Duke University Press.

4. Taussig, Michael. 1993. *Mimesis and Alterity: A Particular History of Senses*. London: Routledge.

5. Mukharji, Projit Bihari. 2009. *Nationalizing the Body, the Medical Market, Print and Daktari medicine*. London: Anthem Press.

6. Quaiser, 2011. op. cit.

7. Quaiser, 2000. op. cit.; "For Muslim Medical Culture"; Quaiser, Neshat. 2001 (a). "Child in Muslim Medical Culture: A Case of Indian Sub-Continent," unpublished. See Abstract in *Book of Abstracts*, EAHMH 5th Conference, 2001.

8. Quaiser, 2011. op. cit.

9. For the notion of Medical Public Sphere in colonial India, see Quaiser, Neshat. 2001 (b), "*Medical Public Sphere* in Colonial India: Competing Meaning Systems of Western and Unani Medicine," unpublished. Paper presented at the Conference on Imperialism, Medicine and South Asia: A Socio Political Perspective, 1800–1950, Cambridge, 14–16 June 2001.

10. Quaiser, Neshat. 2001 (c). "Politics, Culture, and Colonialism: Unani's Debate with Doctory." In *Health, Medicine, and Empire: Perspectives on Colonial India*, edited by Biswamoy Pati and Mark Harrison. Hyderabad: Orient Longman.

11. Quaiser, 2011. op. cit.

12. Awfi, Nuruddin Muhammad. 1906. *Lubab al-Albab*, vol. 2: Leiden Brill, 127.

13. Quaiser, 2001c.

14. For a discussion on the notion of parallel practice see Quaiser, Neshat. 1994. "Some Reflections [on Parallel Practice]," *Seminar* 423 (November).

15. For influential discussions on memory, the past, and representation see Halbwacs, Maurice. 1950. *On Collective Memory*. Chicago: University of Chicago Press; Shils, Edward. 1975. *Centre and Periphery: Essays in Macrosociology*. Chicago: University of Chicago Press; Eliade, Mircea. 1963. *Myth and Reality*. New York: Harper and Row; Hobsbawm, E. J., and Ranger, Terence. 1983. *The Invention of Tradition*. Cambridge: Cambridge University Press; Nora, Pierre, and Le Goff, Jacquese, eds. 1985. *Constructing the Past*. Cambridge: Cambridge University Press; Bond, George C., and Gilliam, Angela, eds. 1994. *Social Construction of the Past: Representation as Power*. London: Routledge; Antez, Paul, and Lambek, Michael, eds. 1996. *Tense Past: Cultural Essays in Trauma and Memory*. London: Routledge; Terdiman, Richard. 1985. "Deconstructing Memory: On Representing the Past and Theorizing Culture in France since the Revolution," *Diacritics* (Winter).

16. For a theoretical discussion on the issue see Cohn, Bernard S. 1996. *Colonialism and Its Forms of Knowledge: The British in India*. Princeton: Princeton University Press. Foreword in Cohn, Bernard S. 1996. *Colonialism and its Forms of Knowledge: The British in India*. Princeton: Princeton University Press; Cooper, Fredrick, and Stoler. Ann Laura, ed. 1977. *Tensions of Empire: Colonial Cultures in a Bourgeois World*. Berkeley: University of California; Irschick, Eugene. 1994. *Dialogue and History: Constructing India, 1795–1895*. Berkeley: University of California Press.

17. For Saidian view and its critical appreciation, see Said, Edward. 1978. *Orientalism*. Harmondsworth: Penguin; Ahmad, Aijaz. 1993. "Orientalism and After: Ambivalence and Metropolitan Location in the Work of Edward Said." In *Theory: Classes, Nations, Literatures*. Bombay: Oxford University Press, 1992. Sprinkler, Michael, ed. 1993. *Edward Said: A Critical Reader*. Cambridge: Blackwell.

18. Basalla, George. 1967. "The Spread of Western Science," *Science* 156:611–22; Flemming, Donald. 1964. "Science in Australia, Canada, and the United States: Some Comparative Remarks." In *Proceedings of the 10th International Congress of the History of Science, 1962*. Paris: Hermann, 1988; Headrick, Daniel, ed. 1987. *The Tentacles of Progress: Technology Transfer in the Age of Imperialism*. New York: Oxford University Press; MacLeod, Roy, ed. 2006. "On Visiting the 'Moving Metropolis': Reflections on the Architecture of Imperial Science." In *Scientific Colonialism: A Cross-Cultural Comparison*, edited by Nathan Reingold and Marc Rothenberg. Washington, DC: Smithsonian Institution Press; *Science and the Raj*. Delhi: Oxford University Press; Harrison, Mark. 2005. *Isis*, 96: 56–63.

19. On the question of science and Unani, see Kabīr al-Dīn's extremely important intervention, Kabeeruddin, Hakim Mohammad. 1923. *Ilmi Jung*. Delhi: Daftar Almaseeh. For some more discussion on the issue see Quaiser, 2001 (c), 345–50, op. cit.; Lbeskind, Claudia. 2002. "Arguing Science: Unani *Tibb*, Hakims, and Biomedicine in India, 1900–1950." In *Plural Medicine, Tradition and Modernity, 1800–2000* edited by Waltraud Ernst, 58–75. London: Routledge; Attewell, Guy. 2007. *Refiguring Unani Tibb: Plural Healing in Late Colonial India*. Hyderabad: Orient Longman.

20. For example, Kumar, Deepak. 2006. *Science and the Raj*. Delhi: Oxford University Press, xii.

21. Harrison, Mark. 2005. *Isis* 96: 63

22. For the influence of science developed in the Muslim world on the development of European scientific thought, see Nasr, Syyed Hossein. 1970. *Science and Civilisation in Islam*. New York: New American Library.

23. For example, Leslie, Charles. 1976. *Asian Medical Systems: A Comparative Study*. Delhi: Motilal Banarsidass Publishers; Attewell, Guy. 2007. *Refiguring Unani Tibb: Plural Healing in Late Colonial India*. Hyderabad: Orient Longman.

24. For different types of responses to Western medicine, see Quaiser, 2001c, op. cit and 2011, op. cit.

25. For discussion on renewal, see Quaiser, 2010, op. cit.

26. Habermas, Jurgen. 1989. *The Structural Transformation of the Public Sphere*. Translated by Thomas Burger. Cambridge: Polity Press.

27. For a critical assessement of the nationalist attitude toward Unani, see Quaiser, 2011 op. cit.

28. Quaiser, 2000 op. cit.

29. For other responses see Quaiser, 2001(c), op. cit.

30. Hālī, Altaf Hussain, (1892) 1925. *Musaddas Hali*, University Press, Aligarh.

31. For an internalist and externalist view on science see: Imre Lakatos. 1970. "History of Science and Its Rational Reconstruction." In *Proceedings of the Biennial Meeting of the Philosophy of Science Association*, 91–136, New York: Springer.

32. Quaiser, Neshat. 1998. "Medicine and Public Sphere in Colonial India." In *Summerhill*. (December). Simla: Indian Institute of Advanced Study. Quaiser, 2001(c), op. cit).

33. Allahabad, Akbar. 1992. *Intekhab Akbar Allahabadi*. Delhi: Maktaba-e-Jamia Ltd.

34. Readers would be reminded of the arrogance of Macaulay's infamous Minutes.

35. Unani was considered to be a *shareef pesha* (noble profession), thus, a key structuring principle in opposition to Western medicine was conscience based ethical values and practices traditionally associated with the profession of *tibb*. Unani's ethical values, thus expressed human concerns with cultural and moral trappings and were offered as an answer to pure professionalism, capitalist market-oriented logic of professional ethics, and the profit-making motives of the practitioners of Western medicine, colonial mechanisms of control and domination within the domain of medicine and health (See Quaiser, 2011).

36. Ayurveda means the complete knowledge for long life or science of longevity of life and here it refers to ayurvedic medicine, which is a system of medicine native to India. The earliest literature on Indian medical practice appeared during the mid-second millennium BCE. The Susruta Samhita and Caraka Samhita are great encyclopedias of medicine compiled from various sources from the mid-first millennium BCE to about 500 CE and form foundational works of Ayurveda. Over the following centuries, ayurvedic practitioners developed a number of medicinal preparations and surgical procedures for the treatment of various ailments. During the colonial period, along with Unani, Ayurveda too was victim of colonial politics of medical machinations.

37. Aarzoo Azeemabadi, Md. Abdul Hai. 1915. *Rafeeq-ul Atibba*. 16 May.

38. Dakani, Jogi, and Yar Hakeem Allah. n.d. "Musaddas Dar Azmat-e-Tibb-e-Qadeem." In *All India Vaidic and Unani Tibbi Conference (AIVUTC) Ke Pehle Salana Jalsa—1910, Ki Report*. Lahore: Refah-e-Aam Steam Press.

39. Dakani and Yar, "Mussaddas."

40. Dakani and Yar, "Mussaddas."

41. Firuz al-Dīn Hakim. 1915. *Rumuz-ul Atibba*. Vol. 2. Lahore, 4.

42. Quaiser, 2000, op. cit; 2001(c) op. cit; Attewell, 2007, op. cit.

43. Quaiser, 2000, op. cit.; 2001(c) op. cit.

44. Individuals who are widely known to the public and whose lifestyle and ideology are the subject of great scrutiny; in the present context they represented the interest of Unani.

45. Jīlani, Ghulam. 1913. *Tareekh-ul Atibba*. Lahore: Nawal Kishore Press, 21; Quaiser, 2001(c), op. cit.

46. In Hussain, Asghar. Written between 1890–1892. *Bahas Mwazna Tibb-e-Doctory Wa Unani*, 21. Delhi.
47. Ahmad, Nazīr. Lecture given at the meeting to inaugurate Madrasa-e-Tibbiya, Delhi (1889). In Ahmad, Deputy Nazīr. 1918. *Likčaron Ka Majmū'a*, 1:177. Agra: Mufīd-e-'ām Steam Press.
48. In Hussain, 1890–1892, 203. op. cit.
49. Hussain, 1890–1892, 203.
50. See Jīlani, 1913, op. cit.
51. See Jīlani, 1913, op. cit.
52. Khān, Ajmal. n.d. *All India Vaidic and Unani Tibbi Conference (AIVUTC) Ke Pehle Salana Jalsa—1910, Ki Report*. Lahore: Refah-e-Aam Steam Press, 96.
53. Abul Qāsim Zuhravi (b 936), the Spanish physician, is well-known for his book on surgery with illustration of surgical instruments.
54. Dakani and Yar, n.d., op.cit.
55. Dakani and Yar, n.d., op.cit.
56. Quaiser, 2011, op. cit.; 2001(c): 345–50, op. cit.
57. Quaiser, 2011, op. cit. on *Hindustanī Dawakhana*, *Zenana Madrasa*, and *Zenana Shifakhana*.
58. *Mujjala-e Tibbiya*. October 1905.
59. *Awadh Akhbaar*. 31 May 1889, in Quaiser, 2000.
60. *Awadh Akhbar*. 13 January 1891.
61. See Quaiser, 1994.

Chapter Nine

Malarial Fever in Nineteenth-Century Bengal

Revisiting the Prophylactic Intervention

Arabinda Samanta

Malarial fever has never been an unknown ailment in Bengal. It accompanied her people from cradle to coffin over a long trajectory of her historical experience. Her acquaintance with this disease can indeed be dated back to the Vedic past. The Bengalis did suffer from fever, and the village *kavirajas* used to prescribe palliative drugs in individual cases. Unable to cope with the medicine they had at their disposal, people had learned to live with it. Nevertheless, malaria never posed a threat to the community for it never appeared with an epidemic vengeance. There is hardly any evidence to show that the disease had ever been an epidemic prior to the British colonial intervention. But Bengal under the British rule offers a different story altogether. Bengal experienced a spate of epidemic malaria throughout the nineteenth and early twentieth centuries. It afflicted a larger number of people on a wider geographical scale. Worse still, it lingered longer over more than a century; malarial fever was transformed into an epidemic, catching the population completely unaware.

This dramatic transformation of the incidence of the disease raises several pertinent questions. First, how did the government react to the appalling specter of death and devastation caused by malaria? What did the colonial government do to arrest its progress? Was it adequately responsive to the emergent situation? What was the nature of its medical intervention? And secondly, how did the local population react to government responses to malaria? Were they critical about the acts of omission and commission of the government? Did they try to "subvert" the official attempt to ameliorate the situation? How did they respond to the epidemic itself? Did they "contest" the colonial intervention by resorting to their indigenous method of controlling the epidemic?

"FEVER": A CONTESTED CATEGORY

There has been a spur in literature on malaria, noticeably more in recent years. Arnold, in his work on malaria and tribal India, reminds us that colonial medical and topographical texts repeatedly identified "fever" as a primary attribute of the environment.[1] Klein has revived our interest in malaria and mortality in Bengal through his painstaking research on the subject.[2] Marking the Madras presidency as his entry point, Muraleedharan has made some significant observations on the colonial government's response to changing medical views.[3] Some recent scholars have questioned the very notion of "malaria," arguing that in the second half of the nineteenth century in Bengal "a malarial epidemic" presented itself as a flexible medical metaphor. Medical professionals, it has been argued, frequently invoked the term "malaria" to explain multiple varieties of physical ailment in a body.[4] There have also been some attempts to engage malaria environmentally while trying to explain its recurrence in colonial Bengal.[5] More recently, scholars have also tried to invest various meanings with the term "malaria" in nineteenth-century Bengal.[6] All these works are important in their own way, contributing to the vast corpus of knowledge on the subject. But the historical trajectory of malarial fever in Bengal and its negotiation by colonial and also by indigenous medical intervention has not yet been adequately addressed.

PROGNOSIS OF THE DISEASE

A brief trajectory of the epidemic of malaria will be an appropriate start for a discussion on the background of the disease. The epidemic began with a devastating career in Bengal. It broke out first at Muhammadpur in Jessore district sometime in the 1820s.[7] It attacked Nadia district in 1832–1833 and devastated the flourishing hamlet of Ula in 1856. It reached Chakda in 1857 and affected the villages on the east bank of the river Hooghly in 24 Parganas from 1859 to 1861. The epidemic crossed the river from Chakda to Tribeni, Bansberia, and the villages north of Bandel in 1857–1859. The fever reached Pandua in 1862 and Dwarbasini in 1863, and spread along the Kana Nadi in 1864.[8] It reached Kana Damodar in 1866 and the east bank of the river Damodar in 1867. It took about ten years to cross the area lying between the Hooghly and the Damodar. It spread across Arambag *thana*, or police station, on the east bank of the Dwarakeswar in 1868 and traversed Goghat *thana* during the next three years. The west bank of the Hooghly in Serampore subdivision was badly affected in 1871–1873. Altogether the epidemic fever visited Hooghly district for about twenty years from 1857 to 1877. Burdwan district was first affected in 1866. Its intensity and ravages were so alarming that in official correspondences, the epidemic was often called "Burdwan Fever." The epidemic spread from Pandua to the village of Ghose, near Memari, and affected the district for about ten years; it spread to Ghatal, in Midnapur district, in 1868. The widespread destruction continued well until 1877.[9]

Almost all the districts of Bengal experienced the epidemic with varying degrees of virulence. It started relaxing its grip in the 1880s. But the respite was short-lived. From the 1890s until the outbreak of World War II, malarial fever became endemic in Bengal. During its heyday, malaria epidemics killed many. Many large households which could boast of thirty to forty members were left, perhaps, with one solitary occupant; whole *mohullahs* and streets had been deserted and large villages, which formerly could hold residents by the thousands, were then reduced to hundreds.[10]

How did the government react to the abrupt proliferation of malaria and the consequent mortality? This apparently simple question defies an easy answer. Its approach to the epidemic was not uniform, nor did its attitude remain constant over the years. One can notice at times contradictory strands in its attitude toward the disease itself as also to the people. The initial response of the government was palliation rather than prevention. Steps were taken to afford some medical relief. The government appointed native doctors, and distributed conventional medicines to diminish the fever. But as the epidemic showed no sign of abatement, Dr. Elliot, a special officer, was deputed in 1862 to visit the affected areas.[11] Dr. Elliot sought to locate its etiology at the rurality, and as such, traveled around the districts of Nadia and Hooghly, and submitted a detailed report on 18 March 1863. He traced the progress of the epidemic from Jessore and Nadia to Hooghly and Burdwan, and explained the various predisposing and exciting causes of its proliferation. The predisposing causes, he argued, helped an ordinary epidemic fever to become a scourge. He attributed its excessive virulence to unventilated houses, unclean tanks overgrown with various noxious weeds, and to the tangled growth of jungle and rank vegetations "with which the Bengali loves to surround and to obscure his dwelling."[12] As regards the causes, Dr. Elliot remarked that the fever was "endemic, becoming epidemic." The causes, he argued, were probably a "specific poison" introduced into the system, most likely through the lungs. He looked for its origin either in exhalation, or secretions from the bodies of those previously affected with the same disease or in malarious emanations rising under peculiar circumstances from certain parts of the earth's surface.

Dr. Elliot's views on the origin of the epidemic was accepted by many. Dr. J. Sutherland, deputy inspector of General of Hospitals, Presidency Circle, argued in 1868 that the prosperous premodern town of Gaur was depopulated in a similar way. He referred to instances of such an epidemic of relapsing fever having occurred in the Patna district in 1856.[13] To Dr. R. F. Thomson, civil assistant surgeon of Hooghly, the fever was largely due to "contaminated drinking water, superabundant vegetations, obstructed drainage surface and wanton human excrement running into them."[14] Dr. D. B. Smith, the sanitary commissioner of Bengal, argued that the disease was not one which merely came at intervals and then disappeared altogether. "It was always present," he insisted, and this was due more or less to local causes which refused to disappear. "The people," he argued, "are to be blamed for their own apathy and impudence, and they are accessory to a great part of their own misery."[15] Dr. Smith further argued that the health of the province depended much on the varying moods of its rivers, especially on their drying up and disappearance. Given a stagnant, foul, shallow, and perhaps half-dried water-way, one might generally expect to find in the persons residing nearby a great state of debility, sickness, spleen diseases, and short life.

Such instances of attributing locality to the ailment and proximity to river or lack of it can be multiplied. Government doctors believed that the immediate cause of the fever was to be sought for in the overcrowded villages, filthy dwellings, closed and confined air of the dense jungles, and decaying vegetable matters. They sought to prove that the fever was an endemic phenomenon, inherent in the very morphology of the province. In other words, they tried to make an ecological construction of the disease.

The question of contagion was, however, discussed at some length, presumably, because it warranted an increasing possibility of infection among the army population and the European civilians. Only three major observers considered the fever to be contagious: Doctors Sutherland, Vercherie, and Jackson. Dr. Vercherie considered the fever to be typhus, traveling slowly through districts much exposed to and suffering from aguish disease. Dr. Jackson believed that the fever had acquired contagious properties, either in Jessore or in Nadia. For him, it was a contagious malarious fever, and he called it "typhomalarial" fever. Those who maintained that it was essentially a malarial fever seldom discussed the question of contagion. The fact that it was malarious was enough to rule out the possibility of contagion.

PATHOLOGY OF THE GOVERNMENT MIND

Contagious or otherwise, the fact that the epidemic traveled from one place to another alarmed the government, lest it should attack the military cantonment and European population. Since the European civilians were concentrated in the town of Calcutta, attempts were made to insulate the British population in the town from the ravages of fever.[16] The concern of the government was understandable. It was especially pressing because of the very high mortality rate among the European soldiers. It has been computed that about one-tenth of the British troops perished in Northern India between 1817 and 1831.[17] This provoked the government to take active measures in handling it. In 1864, presidency sanitary commissions were set up to help in matters relating to the health of the army, and to supervise the gradual introduction of sanitary improvement in barracks, hospitals, and stations on a continuing basis.[18] But the colonial government was least concerned about the impact of malaria epidemic on the indigenous civil population. The prevailing attitude of the government during the epidemic years can be best understood from the general observation of Whinfield, the Magistrate of Burdwan:

> Can Government do anything to mend mattes? I think not. The people here will not emigrate, and when that is said, no opening appears to remain for Government interference. . . . the people will infallibly populate on and press harder and harder on the means of subsistence as their fathers did before them, till they get a check in the shape of Burdwan fever, or famine, which will again reduce population within the limits which the district can support.

The Magistrate concluded that "Nature is stronger than Government, and there is no use in trying to fight against her laws."[19] Despite such premonitions in some quarters, the government decided to act to protect its revenue, for a morbid rural population might compromise its revenue return. It complied with the recommendations of Dr. Elliot and resorted to the removal of superabundant trees, shrubs, bamboo clumps, and plantation groves from the immediate vicinity of houses. Government officials started pruning and thinning of trees. They removed trees and bamboos from the sides of village tanks. Low busy jungles were uprooted and burnt. Vegetations and rank grasses were weeded out. Larger tanks were deepened and cleansed. The government filled in abandoned tanks, water courses, and other excavations in various neighborhoods. It asked the villagers to set aside particular tanks exclusively for the supply of drinking water. Besides, drains were constructed and roads were built in villages. Burial grounds and burning *ghats* were maintained carefully.[20] Through these measures during the initial years of the epidemic ravages, the government hoped to mitigate the fever. But its hopes were belied. The fever continued to engulf village after village. In some places, it relapsed with greater degree of virulence. In effect, the measures adopted by the government were selective, piecemeal, and perfunctory. A comprehensive program for the eradication of malaria called for a huge medical investment and creation of a special agency, neither of which the government was prepared to undertake. As early as 1863, the Commissioner of Nadia pleaded that judicious expenditure, however large, would save not only the inhabitants of the suffering villages, but would "defend from its ravages the troops at Barrackpore and Dum Dum, and the inhabitants of Calcutta itself."[21] The government was perturbed by these warnings, but its response was tardy; it sanctioned only ten thousand rupees to achieve this enormous task.[22] It pinned its hope to private initiatives.[23] The lieutenant governor openly declared that he could not expend any sum of money from the general revenue of the state in "remedying the condition to which the people of a particular part of the country have reduced themselves by apathy and neglect."[24]

By the beginning of 1870, the government implemented a new scheme for medical relief to the ailing districts, each of which was divided into specified geographical areas to facilitate medical aid. While the existing hospitals and medical establishments were equipped with medical technology to deal with medical issues, new ones were established simultaneously. The expenses were, however, met from special funds, donations, and subscriptions, and were rarely supplemented from the revenue of the state.

TRAJECTORY OF GOVERNMENT AMBIVALENCE

The trajectory of changing prophylactic intervention by the government toward the epidemic fever in colonial Bengal may be summed up in three phases. One, the government initiated a program of environmental improvement including pruning trees and jungles; two, the state-sponsored sanitation measures; and three, its provision of relief in the form of food, medical aid, and doctors to the affected villages. Efforts to clean the local environment entailed monetary expenses apart from deployment of men to do the job. The government sought to solve the problem of money by taking recourse to compulsory subscription from villagers. In most cases, medical bureaucrats would call on village notables and threaten to invoke penal laws if conditions of the villages were not improved by self-help.[25] Large trees, branches, and jungles were, indeed, cleared by the orders of magistrates, but those were not removed or burned out. The result was that during the rainy season, the fallen tress decayed and caused unhealthy living conditions prone to more illness.[26] Besides, little discretion was applied to the felling of trees. Large trees were indiscriminately cut down. Sometimes, fruit-bearing trees like mango, coconut, or jack fruit were mercilessly grounded. Large palmyra and date-palm trees were also not spared. They were pulled down by the coolies of the Public Works Department. Of all the districts, Jessore was the worst sufferer in this respect. The government argued that in many cases the loss fell not on the lower classes who rented them, but upon the landlords who owned them. It was argued that the *raiyats* could expect some remission of their rents from the landlords. But the government seemed to have ignored the fact that most of the Bengali households had grown trees of their own around their homesteads. And so the question of remission of rent became irrelevant.

In addition, notices were served on the villagers to clean their lands within twenty-four to forty-eight hours. Such short-time notices, the villagers argued, were "definitely scanty allowances." The government brushed aside such allegation by arguing that notices were seldom issued "till sufficient time had elapsed and the receiver had shown by his indifference that he was unworthy of further consideration or indulgence."[27] It was unfortunate that the government interpreted the alleged "indifference" as an indication of the *raiyats*' insubordination. The colonial officials refused to understand that the even tenor of Bengal countryside was completely shattered by the sudden intervention of malaria epidemic. Attending to an ailing inmate in the household was certainly their priority. They pleaded that the working hands had been drastically reduced and the rest were too weak to help themselves. It is certainly true that a crisis like this necessitated prompt action and that some inconveniences and losses were unavoidable, but the highhanded attitude of the government officials caused deep resentment among the villagers.

In the meantime, harrowing reports of people's misery started pouring in; and interestingly, the reports of public woe came from their own conscientious medical bureaucrats themselves. Conditions of the people in the affected districts were reported to be "to the last degree pitiable" and that it was quite unlikely to "meet a healthy man."[28] Hundreds had already died, many houses were abandoned. Even those who were able to walk were care-worn and cadaverous. Plaintive women were found imploring passersby for relief. Women and children, on the last stage of attenuation, were seen everywhere with none around to cook food for them, to offer them water, or provide them help.

Such reports were unpalatable to the government. Dr. Smith was, therefore, often accused by his superiors of "over-coloring and of sentimental misrepresentation." Undaunted, Dr. Smith tried to convince the government that there were thousands whose lives were likely to be saved if only efficient medical relief was afforded on a systematic and extended scale. The government felt compelled to shed its ambivalence and adopt more meaningful schemes. Medical and food-relief measures were adapted as succor to the sick and to lessen mortality. But the funds allocated for the purpose were inadequate. The government depended largely on local subscriptions and the benevolence of the Maharaja of Burdwan. In addition to medical and food relief, the sanitary commissioner suggested the improvement in drainage and water supply, reclamation of waste lands, deepening of tanks, and raising of municipal loans. The government acted upon some of his recommendations keeping in mind the disproportionate number of medical relief centers against the number of people afflicted. Dr. Smith's proposal to the government stating that by such measures "agricultural industry would receive a fresh impetus, the resource of the district would be multiplied, and revenue would accrue, in large amount, to the state,"[29] convinced the government for quick decisions on the issue. As a result, food depots were opened up by the government along with new dispensaries in Burdwan and Hooghly. But the food depots were neither provided with adequate food nor were the charitable fever dispensaries equipped with medicines or qualified doctors. By the time fever ravaged Burdwan and Hooghly and entered newer districts like Midnapur and Birbhum, the government had exhausted the available supply of medical subordinates.[30] Relief centers very often ran short of food. Some of the dispensaries were not suitably located and were inaccessible during rains. Interior villages could hardly be reached due to transport problems. Elephants were tried out by the inspecting doctors, but the traveling allowances approved by the government were too small to maintain too large an animal.

The lukewarm response and perfunctory intervention of the government against malarial fever in Bengal stood in sharp contrast to its swift and drastic action against the plague epidemic in Bombay in 1896. By that time contagionism had been firmly established as a theory and was in full control of medical policy in India. Plague was identified as an invading disease, probably imported by sea from Hong Kong, and not a "native malady" originating from within its environmental specificities. It threatened the commercial life of India's second largest port and manufacturing center. The official response was, therefore, prompt and vigorous. Pilgrimages and fairs were stopped, and travelers by roads and rails were examined for signs of plague. Compulsory hospitalization was enforced, clothing and bedding was fumigated or burned. Suspected dwellings were evacuated or broken open to improve ventilation. Most importantly, mass inoculation became a central feature of the anti-plague campaign.[31] But strikingly enough, this sense of urgency was lacking in the anti-malaria campaign in Bengal. The reasons are, however, not far to seek. Malaria was not a contagious disease. Though the subject of the contagious property of malaria was hotly debated, its non-contagious nature was conclusively proved in the last decade of the nineteenth century by Ronald Ross's intervention.[32] Besides, malaria, unlike plague and cholera, was less drastic, less dramatic, and less spectacular in its impact. It was certainly a killer disease, but the act of killing was neither instantaneous nor so drastic as plague or cholera to warrant fear and urgency.

Issues of providing medical relief were best responded to for the army,[33] which remained the main concern for the British administration. The question of fever deaths among British soldiers could not be ignored as a result. Epidemics created the most compelling predicament to their war efforts. The incidence of malaria was of a still greater importance in war, for it often incapacitated more troops than battle casualties. Many a time military operations had been stalled by malaria. During the Rangoon Expedition of 1804–1805, there were only thirty-five deaths from wounds, but 450 out of one thousand men engaged died of malaria. In the Burma Expedition of 1824, the enterprise in Arakan had to be abandoned owing to fever, for every one who was not dead was in hospital (75 percent of the whole force in action). During World War I in Macedonia, there were 1,62,517 admissions to hospitals for malaria among the British troops as compared with 23,762 battle casualties. The story was repeated during World War II. In 1942, a quarter of the force in the Assam front suffered from a small-winged enemy—the Anopheles minimus.[34] Field Marshal Lord Wavell instructed the GOCs-in-C that "in theaters where future operations are likely to take place may well find that disease, and especially malaria, is a more dangerous factor than enemy resistance."[35]

ANATOMY OF THE POPULAR MIND

In Bengal, most deities were associated with a particular disease or ailment. Her principal deity was *Sitala*, the goddess of smallpox. The worship of *Sitala* was timed to coincide with the beginning of the smallpox season.[36] In deltaic Bengal, the specific cholera deity was called *Ola Bibi* by the Muslims and *Olai Chandi* by the Hindus.[37] But interestingly, malaria was hardly ever interpreted as a disease caused by heavenly intervention. Consequently, one finds no socially acclaimed folk deity for fever epidemic, excepting, of course, the cult of *jwarasura* prevalent among the lower classes of people. Some marginalized social caste groups generally invoked *jwarasura*, the fever demon, with the help of a Brahmin during epidemic malaria to get rid of fever in individual as well as community affliction.[38] Apart from the usual offerings of rice, sweets, and fruits, goats were sacrificed in special instances. But *jwarasura* seems to have had no following among the upper-caste Hindus or the well-to-do villagers. For nowhere in the contemporary literary works or in the official records could one find any reference to a universal worship of this particular deity. In other words the disease deity, unlike *Sitala* or *Ola Bibi*, never became a cult in Bengali society. The explanation for this is twofold: lack of indigenous immunity, and an exceptional geographical range. First, Bengalis, until the beginning of the twentieth century, did not know the causes of malarial fever, and quinine, its herbal remedy, remained relatively unknown. People sought solace in the popular adage: that which cannot be ended should be mended, and which could not even be mended should be accommodated within the social milieu.[39] Moreover, malarial fever can be remittent or intermittent. Its nature of periodic invasion provided the patient temporary respite from fever providing temporary relief. Familiarity with the experience of the ailment also helped reduce the fear from it. Second, epidemic malaria lost much of its edge due to its widespread spatial expansion. It was not an isolated ailment, afflicting a particular person or two. It traveled from Amritsar to Assam, from Bombay to Bengal. In Bengal, in particular, few districts could escape its ravages. The epidemic became almost a pan-Indian phenomenon, visiting multiple sites simultaneously. Thus, the element of fear diminished, with an attitude of helpless resignation either to conventional treatment or to fate. Arguably, therefore, since the epidemic was scarcely regarded as a sign of divine displeasure, the need to worship or propitiation of a particular deity was not pressed upon.

On the contrary, people accused the colonial government of arbitrary interference with the river system in eastern India and consequently setting off the epidemic fever. Railway embankments, people argued, had converted large tracts of fertile land into perpetual swamps.[40] Increasing numbers of embankments and railways reduced the chances of flood and inundations, and reduced chances of flood meant progressive loss of fertility of the soil. The consequences, people argued, were generally twofold. First, impeded drainage brought in its trail a large number of stagnant pools and vegetated marshes, which provided congenial breeding grounds for mosquitoes. Second, loss of fertility of the soil due to cessation of inundation had diminished the amount of winter harvest, which meant starvation for a sizeable section of the rural masses. The government was seen as uninterested in bringing the rivers to their functional regimes.

If the people lamented over the acts of omission, they protested against the rulers' acts of commission as well. Since many of the affected villages were particularly overgrown with tangled vegetations, government officials decried its growth in the immediate vicinity of the dwelling houses. The government may have been well intentioned, but some of the overzealous officials resorted to measures, which virtually denuded the villages of the lush green. They chopped off branches of trees, cut down the shrubs short, and worse still, uprooted the larger trees, particularly the fruit-bearing ones.

Such alleged official high-handedness never went unprotested. People in the affected areas, particularly in Jessore, were up in arms when the government officials approached the villages with their men to execute the government orders. The officials entrusted with the unpleasant task had to beat hasty retreat, lamenting that villagers had displayed much apathy to their own welfare, and in some cases "even offered resistance to measures solely adopted for their benefit."[41] They also encountered similar resistance from villagers when the government opened up *langarkhana*, or gruel kitchens, in the neighborhood of affected villages. When the government introduced relief-houses first at Burdwan, people were opposed to the system of giving cooked food on religious grounds, and sarcastically called it "hotel."[42] The Hindus did not approve of cooked food being distributed, especially the upper caste Hindus for whom it was preposterous to join the pack of alms-receivers. Each individual was furnished with a printed ticket, which entitled him or her to receive the stipulated amount of food relief. The recipients, it was admitted by the government officials, generally consisted of the lower caste people, mostly women and children of humble social status.[43] Nevertheless, the Muslims seemed to have had no inhibitions with cooked food, for at least at one depot at Nilpur they were very keen to receive the relief provided by the *langarkhana*.[44]

Elements of popular protest to sanitation measures in terms of cutting of trees were, thus, noticeable. Opposition to the provision of food relief was also discernable. But opposition to government dispensaries was seldom noticed. The government opened up "fever hospitals" and fever dispensaries in the affected areas, which provided quinine free of cost to the ailing villagers. Initially, people seemed to be rather indifferent to such medical institutions, partly because the doctors in charge were mostly unconcerned with treatment and irregular in their attendance. In some places, the government doctors were allegedly taking fees for medical advice.[45] Gradually, however, these institutions became very popular and an increasing number of patients started queuing before the outdoor departments.[46]

The intensity of malarial fever and the consequent hospitalization of the afflicted, thus, evoked little or no resistance from the masses. This stood out in sharp contrast to the phenomenon of plague epidemic in Bombay. The physical examination of travelers and the residents of plague-struck towns and cities, hospitalization, and segregation, produced tremendous alarm among the masses, and they opposed the measures tooth and nail.[47] Because most of the inspecting doctors were male as well as European, mere touch by them was considered either polluting, or tantamount to sexual molestation, particularly when it involved the examination of women's necks, armpits, and thighs. Arnold relates the repugnance of the oriental bodies to Western medicine for religious and social reasons, their loud protest against subjection of the native body to European doctors' inspection, and, finally, the mitigation of harsh government measures to placate the turbulent circumstances.[48] Nothing of this sort happened in Bengal when, initially, the Company and then the Crown resorted to some sort of social segregation for mitigating the epidemic fever by way of internment in hospitals and doling out Western medicine through public distribution systems such as dispensaries and post offices.

Arguably, the explanation may be twofold. First, in the case of plague, people considered it as an expression of divine wrath. The Indians saw plague as a form of divine punishment, a visitation against which the use of Western medicine was bound to be either impious or ineffective. But malaria, unlike plague, was never interpreted as a divine intervention, far less a punishment by the heavenly hand. In collective imagination, its virulence was associated with the baneful effects of British colonial policy. People argued that since the government had stirred up the disease, none but the government would take up the responsibility of remedying the situation. Second, treatment of malarial fever with indigenous medicine generally proved ineffective. Thousands died even without any treatment at all. In most cases, death was hastened by "injudicious treatment from ignorant and unqualified native practitioners."[49] Government officials believed that the unabated mortality was due primarily to wrong treatment by the *kavirajas*, and people as such were increasingly losing faith in their treatment.[50] At the same time, people admitted the efficacy of European medicines in sharp contrast to the "uncertain" cure under the indigenous systems. Yet, when the epidemic fever first struck the Bengal countryside in the 1860s, people were filled with dismay. Initially, the epidemic did not prove fatal, although gradually malarial fever spread to several districts killing some and debilitating others. People had never seen so many people die in such short spells in their villages. Funeral processions with the ritual chanting of *Hari* stalked the countryside everyday. The funeral pyres, it seemed, at the burning ghats were never put out; when mortal remains of one person were reduced to ashes, those of another were ready for cremation. Elderly inhabitants confessed that they had never seen such a terrible visitation. From nearly every house, the cry of lamentation could be heard.[51] Only when the government started sending out native doctors trained in Western medicine and opened up charitable dispensaries did the pervasive public fear gradually subside.[52]

Available evidence indicates that the poor peasant families refused to move out of their homesteads to other healthier districts even in periods of high malaria mortality. Government officials could hardly induce the villagers to leave their family residence, the *bhadrasanbati*, in which were installed the family deities and which was supposedly guarded by the spirits of their deceased ancestors.[53] Migration to healthier places, particularly to Calcutta, the capital city, was, however, very common among the well-to-do families, especially among the zamindars. The attitude of the better-off peasants, smaller zamindars, and other wealthy influentials to the fever epidemic was more or less practical, and the methods they evolved to circumvent it seemed pragmatic. They were not necessarily fatalist, and they did not worship *jwarasura* either. They used to call on the village *vaidyas* or *kavirajas*, failing which they looked for better cures. Quite often, they would visit the government dispensaries attended by native doctors practicing Western medicine. If none of these worked, as the last resort, they would leave the affected village for good and settle in the city. This was more or less common with the zamindars.[54]

When the government resorted to cleaning the jungles in an attempt to destroy the habitat of mosquitoes, the better off and more influential natives proved to be the worst troubleshooters. They were opposed to the sanitary operations and tried to incite the villagers to stop implementation of these operations.[55] Conspicuous among them was the manager of Prasanna Kumar Tagore's property which the government officials believed was instrumental in manipulating the local population for opposition.[56] There were, of course, some exceptions. The Maharaja of Burdwan and Jaykrishna Mukherjee of Uttarpara did come forward to help the local people. Yet, most of the Bengal zamindars were apathetic to the general welfare of their *raiyats*. They had neither the inclination nor the means to undertake these works, owing to a dwindling income from their land under the revised revenue demands by the government from time to time.

A few tentative conclusions can be drawn from all of these. Response to the malaria epidemic from different sections of the society followed neither a homogenous nor a unilinear trajectory. "Fragmentations" stemmed from their widely differential perceptions about the epidemic itself. Generally speaking, the response of the masses was one of stoic acceptance, and not a dreaded repulsion. There is, however, nothing new in this kind of attitude, for an epidemic such as this had never been a dreaded phenomenon in Bengal. It has all along been depicted in Bengali folklore as a living entity, often described as a "cute village belle who delights in frequenting village huts, and although often despised by the wealthy landlords, is invited by the impoverished peasants." On a general note, reaction to the prophylactic intervention by the government became rigid over a period of time. It followed more or less a uniform pattern everywhere with marginal variations. Almost all sections of the society looked at the colonial government and the policies with suspicion and disbelief. The accusation was sometimes violent, sometimes muted. Reputed doctors held the rulers responsible for the epidemic, while blaming the people for their apathy to personal health and hygiene. They constructed the epidemic from a purely medical perception, which was an error in judgment. They could have realized that the struggle against disease must begin with a war against bad government.

It is true that prophylactic intervention against malarial fever in nineteenth-century Bengal had some limitations. Lack of appropriate epidemiological knowledge was the most plausible cause, but the colonial situation cannot be ignored either. Apart from difficulties in creating an appropriate mass-immunization agency that would suit the culture of the people, the very nature of the colonial regime reinforced the cultural distance. Disposed to see the health of its own European subjects as its priority, the colonial state was reluctant to make the financial commitment necessary for effectively combating malaria. In retrospect, although the intensity of health and medical matters may have reinforced lack of initiatives, the effect of ensuing competition within the medical profession and the difficult sociocultural barriers can hardly be denied because, after all, medical facilities were limited to a few.

NOTES

1. David Arnold, "Disease, Resistance and India's Ecological Frontier, 1770–1947." Pp. 1–22 in *Issues in Modern Indian History*, edited by Biswamoy Pati (Mumbai: Popular Prakashan, 2000).
2. Ira Klein, "Malaria and Mortality in Bengal, 1840–1921." *Indian Economic and Social History Review* 9, no. 2 (1972).
3. V. R. Muraleedharan, "Malady in Madras: The Colonial Government's Response to Malaria in the Early Twentieth Century." Pp. 101–112 in *Science and Empire: Essays in Indian Context*, edited by Deepak Kumar (New Delhi: Anamika Prakashan, 2001).
4. Rohan Deb Roy, "'An Unseen Awful Visitant': The Making of Burdwan Fever." *Economic and Political Weekly* 43, no. 12–13 (2008): 62–70.
5. Ihtesham Kazi, "Environmental Factors Contributing to Malaria in Colonial Bengal." In *Disease and Medicine in India: A Historical Overview*, edited by Deepak Kumar (New Delhi: Tulika, 2001); Sujata Mukherjee, "Environmental Thoughts and Malaria in Colonial Bengal: A Study in Social Response." *Economic and Political Weekly* 43, no. 12–13 (2008): 54–61.
6. Rohan Deb Roy, "Mal-areas of Health: Dispersed Histories of a Diagnostic Category." *Economic and Political Weekly,* 42, no. 2 (13 January 2007).
7. M. A. Momen, *Final Report on the Survey and Settlement Operation in the District of Jessore, 1920–1924* (Calcutta: Bengal Secretariat Book Depot, 1925), 19
8. L. S. S. O'Malley, *Bengal District Gazetteers, Jessore* (Calcutta: Bengal Secretariat Book Depot, 1912), 61
9. D. G. Crawford, *Hooghli Medical Gazetteer* (Calcutta: Bengal Secretariat Book Depot, 1903), 113
10. Home Department, Public Branch, 7 May 1870 (New Delhi: National Archives of India), 65–71.
11. C. E. Buckland, *Bengal under the Lieutenant-Governors, Being a Narrative of the Principal Events and Public Measures during Their Periods of Service, from 1854 to 1898,* vol. 1 (Calcutta: S. K. Lahiri and Co., Kolkata, 1901), 290.
12. Proceedings of the Government of Bengal (hereafter Progs. GOB), General Department (hereafter Gen. Dept.) March 1863, no. 108, West Bengal State Archives (hereafter WBSA), 63–64.
13. Progs. GOB, Gen. Dept. Sanitation Branch (hereafter San. Br.) June 1868, no. 14, WBSA.
14. R. F. Thompson, Letter no. 34, 17 March, Progs. GOB, Gen. Dept. San. Br. June 1868, no. 14, WBSA.
15. Progs. GOB, Gen. Dept. San. Br. June 1870, no. 10–12, WBSA.
16. Poonam Bala, *Imperialism and Medicine in Bengal: A Socio-Historical Perspective* (New Delhi: Sage, 1991), 101.
17. Radhika Ramasubban, *Public Health and Medical Research in India: Their Origin under the Impact of British Colonial Policy* (New Delhi: SAREC Report, 1982), 16.
18. Bala, *Imperialism and Medicine in Bengal*, 102
19. D. G. Crawford, *Hooghli Medical Gazetteer* (Calcutta: Bengal Secretariat Press, 1903), 147
20. C. E. Buckland, *Bengal under the Lieutenant-Governors*, 290–91

21. V. H. Schalch, Commissioner of Nadia to the Secretary to the GOB (no. 8ct, dated 13 February 1863). Progs of the GOB, Gen. Dept., March 1863, no. 46, 27, WBSA.
22. S. C. Bayley, Junior Secretary to the GOB, to the Officiating Secretary to the GOB PWD (No. 1482, dated 27 March 1863). Progs of the GOB, Gen. Dept., March 1863, no. 110, 76, WBSA.
23. A. Eden, Secy to the GOB, to A. T. Maclean (no. 1491, dated 30 March 1863). Progs of the GOB. Gen. Dept., March 1863, no. 113, 79, WBSA.
24. A. Eden, Secy to the GOB, to the Honorary Secy to the British India Association (no. 1490, dated 30 March 1863). Progs of the GOB, Gen. Dept., March 1863, no. 112, 76–78, WBSA.
25. J. D. Maclean, Magistrate on Special Duty to A. V. Palmer, Magistrate of Hooghly (no. 21, dated 14 July 1863). Progs of the GOB, Gen. Dept., July 1863, no. 129, 79, Microfilm, Gen. Dept. Roll No. P.170, vol 7. WBSA.
26. W. D. Short, Superintending Engineer, Burdwan Circle, to the Officiating Chief Engineer, Bengal (no. 664, dated 3 July 1863), Microfilm Roll No. P 170, 1863, vol. 7. WBSA.
27. J. D. Maclean, Magistrate on Special Duty to A. V. Palmer, Magistrate of Hooghly (no. 21, dated 14 July 1863). Progs of the GOB, Gen. Dept., July 1863, no. 129, 79, Microfilm, Gen. Dept. Roll no. P.170, 1863, vol 7. WBSA.
28. D. B. Smith, Sanitary Commissioner, Bengal, to C. T. Buckland, Commissioner of the Burdwan Division (no. 4, dated 4 November 1869). Progs of the GOB, Political Department, Medical Branch, December 1869, no. 4, 2. WBSA.
29. D. B. Smith, secretary to the GOB. In the Judicial Department. (Dated Hooghly 25 March 1869). Progs of the GOB, May 1869, General Department, Sanitation Branch, no. 13, 17. WBSA.
30. A. Mackenzie, officiating secretary to the GOB, Judicial Dept. (no. 573, dated Calcutta 21 October 1872) to the commissioner of the Burdwan Division. Progs of the GOB, Gen. Dept., Medical Branch, November 1872, no. 26, 76–77. WBSA.
31. David Arnold, "Cholera and Colonialism in British India." *Past and Present* 113 (1986): 147. Also see David Arnold, "Touching the Body: Perspectives on the Indian Plague, 1896–1900." In *Selected Subaltern Studies,* edited by Ranajit Guha et al. (New Delhi: Oxford University Press, 1988).
32. Arabinda Samanta, "Sir Ronald Ross and Malaria: The Colonial Perspective." Pp. 138–148 in *Explorations in History: Essays in Honour of Prof Chittabrata Palit,* edited Abhijit Dutta et al. (Calcutta: Corpus Research Institute, 2003).
33. Radhika Ramasubban, "Imperial Health in British India." Pp. 38–60 in *Disease, Medicine and Empire: Perspectives on Western Medicine and Experiences of European Expansion,* edited by Roy Macleod et al. (London: Routledge, 1988).
34. G. Covell, "The Prophylaxis and Treatment of Malaria in War." *Journal of the Malaria Institute of India* 5 (1943): 125–29.
35. M. K. Afridi, "Official History of the Indian Armed Forces in the Second World War." *Indian Journal of Malariology* 16, no. 4 (1962): 393.
36. R. W. Nicholas, "The Goddess Sitala and Epidemic Smallpox in Bengal." *Journal of Asian Studies* 41, no. 1 (1981): 21–44.
37. Gopendra Krishna Basu, *Banglar Loukik Devata* (Calcutta: Ananda Publishers, 1964), 25–28, 195–98.
38. L. S. S. O'Malley and Monmohan Chakraborty, *Bengal District Gazetteers, Howrah* (Calcutta: Bengal Secretariat Book Depot, 1909), 46.
39. Instances of such attitude of helpless resignation to fate can be found in abundance in the novels and short stories by Saratchandra Chattopadhyay, the most notable ones being "Pallisamaj," "Panditmasay," and "Datta." In *Sulabh Sarat Samgraha* (Calcutta: Ananda Publishers, 1989), 94, 140, 794.
40. Editorial Comments in *Gramer Daak*, a bi-monthly journal of Howrah Jila Krishak o Hitakari Samiti. Ashar-Sravan, 1334 (B. S.), 20.
41. G. S. Hills, on Special Duty, to the Hon'ble A. Eden, Secy to the GOB. Progs of the GOB, Gen. Dept., August 1863, no. 20. Microfilm Roll no. P 170, vol. 8. WBSA.

42. C. T. Buckland, Officiating Commissioner of the Burdwan Division, to the Secy to the GOB. (no. 80T dated Burdwan, 7 February 1870). Progs of the GOB, Medical Dept. Sanitation Br. Feb. 1870, no. 30, 19–20. WBSA.

43. Buckland, "To the Secy to the GOB."

44. Buckland, "To the Secy to the GOB," 21.

45. R. F. Thompson's Report on the General Result of the Working of Each Dispensary in Hooghly. Progs of the GOB, Political Dept. San Br. May 1870, no. 13, 9–15. WBSA.

46. A Hilton, "Report of the Calcutta Medical Institutions for the Year 1890." Progs of the GOB, Municipal Dept. Medical Br. June 1891, 155, WBSA.

47. David Arnold, "Touching the Body: Perspectives on the Indian Plague, 1896–1900." Pp. 397–401 in *Selected Subaltern Studies*, edited by Ranjit Guha and Gayatri Chakraborty Spivak (New Delhi: Oxford University Press, 1988).

48. Arnold, "Touching the Body," 397–401.

49. Progs of the GOB. Gen. Dept., March 1863. No. 108, 69. WBSA.

50. Progs of the GOB. Gen. Dept., San Br. June 1868. No. 14, 19.WBSA.

51. Rev. Lal Behari Dey, *Bengal Peasant Life* (London: Macmillan and Co., 1878), 250.

52. Bala, *Imperialism and Medicine in Bengal*. 57, 60, 62.

53. Report of R. C. Mukherjee, condensed in Pellow's Report dated 24 March 1878. Cited in Crawford, *Hooghli Medical Gazetteer*, 138.

54. Gurucharan Rakshit, "Pallir Durdasha." *Krishak* 22, no. 5 (1328 BS): 121.

55. G. S. Hill to A. Eden. Progs of the GOB. Gen. Dept., August 1863. Microfilm Roll no. P. 170, vol. 8, no. 41, 20. WBSA.

56. W. D. Short, Superintending Engineer, Burdwan Circle, to the Officiating Chief Engineer, Bengal (no. 664 dated 3 July 1863). Progs of the GOB. Gen. Dept. Med. Br. July 1863, no. 102, 58. Microfilm Roll No. P. 170, vol. 7. WBSA.

Index

About the Contributors

Poonam Bala teaches sociology and is currently a visiting scholar at Cleveland State University, Ohio, prior to which she was a visiting professor at the University of South Africa and associate professor at the Delhi School of Economics, University of Delhi, India. She has published widely on medicine, health, and disease in colonial India. Her recent research on social issues of poverty, history of cancer, and stem cell technology has been published in *Encyclopedia of Cancer* and *Encyclopedia of Stem Cell Technology*. She has authored *Imperialism and Medicine in Bengal* and *Medicine and Medical Policies in India: Social and Historical Perspectives*, and edited *Biomedicine as a Contested Site: Some Revelations in Imperial Contexts*; she is currently working on colonial medical services as well as comparative themes between India and South Africa.

Madhulika Banerjee is associate professor of political science at the University of Delhi, India. She has published widely on various issues in policy in Ayurvedic pharmaceuticals in India, in various journals including *Economic and Political Weekly* and *Contributions to Indian Sociology*. She has authored *Power, Knowledge, Medicine: Ayurvedic Pharmaceuticals at Home and in the World* and edited (with Manisha Priyam and Krishna Menon) *Human Rights: Gender and the Environment*.

Cristiana Bastos is an anthropologist at the Institute of Social Sciences, University of Lisbon, Portugal. She has taught in different graduate programs in Portugal, Brazil, and the United States. Her interests lie at the intersections of society, knowledge, and power. Her recent research on Portuguese colonialism and its health institutions is at the confluence of anthropology, history, and science studies. She is the author of *Global Responses to AIDS: Science* *in Emergency* and a number of articles on topics of colonialism, medicine, and displacement in *Análise Social*, *Etnográfica*, *História*, *Ciências Saúde-Manguinhos*, *Journal of Romance Studies*, *Journal of Southern African Studies*, *International Migration*, *Bulletin of the History of Medicine*, and *Horizontes Antropológicos*. She recently edited the special issue "Parts of Asia" for the journal *Portuguese Literary and Cultural Studies* and coedited "Healing Holidays" for the journal *Anthropology and Medicine*.

Shrimoy Roy Chaudhury is a researcher in history at the Maxwell School of Citizenship and Public Affairs, Syracuse University, New York. He has been a fellow in South and South East Asian Studies at Syracuse University, and has taught in various universities in India. His research focuses on various aspects of locating medical histories, presented at the Wellcome Trust Centre for the History of Medicine (University College London), Jawaharlal Nehru University (Delhi), and at the Wellcome Unit for History of Medicine in Oxford (UK).

Shamshad Khan is a post-doctoral fellow at the CIHR (Canadian Institutes of Health Research) International Infectious Disease and Global Health Training Program Post-Doctoral Fellow at the Centre for Global Public Health, University of Manitoba, Canada. He obtained his doctoral degree in communication at the School of Communication, Simon Fraser University, British Columbia, Canada. He has published in leading academic journals such as *Social Science and Medicine* and *Social Scientist*, and has a wide range of research interests including public health and policy, health, development and social issues in communication, media representation of policy and discourse analysis, social history of disease and medicine, science and public policy, international development and nationalism, and nation-state and governance in postcolonial societies.

Seān Lang is senior lecturer in history at Anglia Ruskin University, Cambridge, UK. He served two terms as honorary secretary of the United Kingdom Historical Association, and has been an adviser to the UK government as well as the Council of Europe on the position of the discipline of history in education. In 2005 he chaired the group that produced the historical association's important report on "History 14–19." His main research focuses on various aspects of women's health in British India, and history of medicine under the British Empire, with published articles in *Social History of Medicine* and *History*. He has also written textbooks including *Parliamentary Reform, 1785–1928* and *Nazi Foreign Policy, 1933–1939*, and is currently working on royal patronage for medical initiatives in India, with focus on the Countess of Dufferin's Fund.

Atsuko Naono is an associate fellow at the Centre for the History of Medicine (Department of History) at the University of Warwick, Warwick, UK. She is also research associate at the Centre for South East Asian Studies at the School of Oriental and African Studies, University of London, UK. She has written extensively on various aspects of public health in colonial Burma, and has special interest in religious and cultural understandings of the body, nongovernmental health organizations, and history of public health. Her major publications include *State of Vaccination*: *The Fight against Smallpox in Colonial Burma*. She has recently been involved with projects ranging from infanticide in nineteenth-century Ireland to transnational health and fitness organizations and their youth wings in colonial Southeast Asia.

Neshat Quaiser is associate professor of sociology at the Jami Millia Islamia University, Delhi, India. He has a wide range of interests including historical sociology of Muslims in the Indian subcontinent, and historical sociology of medicine with reference to Unani and Western medicine. He has written and published widely on aspects of Unani medical culture, medicine under the empire, and postcolonial medicine.

Arabinda Samanta is professor of history at the University of Burdwan, west Bengal, India. He was a visiting fellow at The Wellcome Trust Centre for the History of Medicine at University College, London, UK and visiting professor, Zakir Husain Centre for Educational Studies, Jawaharlal Nehru University, New Delhi. He has written extensively on various aspects of social history of Bengal, with contributions having appeared *inter alia*, in *Economic and Political Weekly*, *Bengal Past and Present*, and *Calcutta Historical Journal*. He has authored *Malarial Fever in Colonial Bengal*: *Social History of an Epidemic*, *Saahityer Itihaas Kimba Itihaaser Saahitya* (Bengali), *Rog, Rogi*, *Raastra*: *Unish Shataker Bangla* (Bengali), *Praatik Biparjay O Manush* (Bengali), and edited *The Revolt of 1857*: *Memory*, *Identity History* and *Life and Culture in Bengal*: *Colonial and Post-Colonial Experiences*. He is currently working on his book, *Locating Epidemics*: *Colonial Bengal, 1820s–1930s*.

www.ingramcontent.com/pod-product-compliance
Ingram Content Group UK Ltd.
Pitfield, Milton Keynes, MK11 3LW, UK
UKHW041627031026
15587UKWH00001B/111

9 780739 170236